"No one in medicine has entered and described the mind and the world of the patient with more clarity than Nortin Hadler, M.D. In *By the Bedside of the Patient*, Dr. Hadler, in his inimitable fashion, places critical thinking, empathetic listening, and evidence-based, mindful care of the patient at the heart of how we must educate the next generation of healers. He applies his critical cognitive filter upon six decades of popular, and at times trendy, educational reform toward the efficient more than the effective, which often drifts away from the compelling patient focus that true care requires. As educators and as practitioners, we need the gift of this book as our anthem for designing the future."
—Stephen Ray Mitchell, Dean for Medical Education, Georgetown University

"Nortin Hadler's book is a brilliant account of the changes in American medicine over the past five decades, which have adversely affected the patient-physician relationship. Dr. Hadler presents innovative solutions to restore medical professionalism in the future."
—Arthur Rubenstein, Raymond and Ruth Perelman School of Medicine, University of Pennsylvania

"In this book, Dr. Hadler reminds us that by the bedside of the patient must be a doctor who cares about the *person*. Medicine can be informed by genomics, proteomics, pharmacogenomics, metabolomics, and epigenomics, but good doctoring is about *personomics*, understanding and appreciating the unique circumstances of every individual cared for."
—Roy Ziegelstein, Sarah Miller Coulson and Frank L. Coulson Jr. Professor of Medicine, Mary Wallace Stanton Professor of Education, and Vice Dean for Education, Johns Hopkins University School of Medicine

By the Bedside of the Patient

By the Bedside of the Patient

LESSONS FOR THE TWENTY-FIRST-CENTURY PHYSICIAN

Nortin M. Hadler, M.D.

The University of North Carolina Press / CHAPEL HILL

The paper in this book meets the guidelines for permanence and durability
of the Committee on Production Guidelines for Book Longevity of the Council on
Library Resources. The University of North Carolina Press has been a member
of the Green Press Initiative since 2003.

Jacket illustration: © Wavebreakmedia, photo i.d. 24055163, istockphoto.com.

Library of Congress Cataloging-in-Publication Data
Hadler, Nortin M., author.
By the bedside of the patient : lessons for the twenty-first-century physician /
Nortin M. Hadler, M.D.
pages cm
Includes bibliographical references and index.
ISBN 978-1-4696-2666-6 (cloth : alk. paper) — ISBN 978-1-4696-2667-3 (ebook)
1. Medical education policy. 2. Patient-centered health care. 3. Medicine—Practice.
I. Title.
R737.H23 2016
610.71—dc23
2015031952

FOR CAROL S. HADLER

Who joined me on this journey fifty years ago and made it ours

Who keeps me grounded

And who provides a "Yes" when I need it most

CONTENTS

FIGURES

ACKNOWLEDGMENTS

The foundation for this book is forty-five years as a practicing physician. But that was not the stimulus for this book. That came from the extraordinary staff of the University of North Carolina Press, who supported me through the publication of my last four books. In the course of the production of the most recent one, *Citizen Patient*, one editor, Jay Mazzocchi, commented that he was surprised to learn that medicine had transformed from a cottage industry to a burgeoning enterprise in the course of only thirty years. Then Gina Mahalek informed me that UNC Press had received correspondence from readers, including physicians in training, asking if I would write a book describing how I, personally, had handled this transition and the pressures it had placed on clinical practice. Jay and Gina pointed out that while *Citizen Patient* renders the current system transparent, it does not explicate how clinical practice and judgment respond to varying sociopolitical constraints. Furthermore, this was not a thesis of the prior four books, which were patient-centered expositions designed to facilitate informed medical decision making by people facing clinical challenges at various stages in life today. This book is my response to the challenge put forward by Jay, Gina, and the correspondents: *By the Bedside of the Patient* is a close look at the patient-physician contract over time. I am grateful for this challenge. It forced me to define sociopolitical pressures that constrain the treatment act. A great many lessons have emerged in this exercise, lessons that surely pertain to the social construction of the treatment act going forward.

The publication process with any university press entails more than acceptability by the editorial staff. Manuscripts are subjected to external "blind peer review" before any manuscript, even one that is written under contract, can be subjected to final review by the editorial staff and the board of directors. *By the Bedside of the Patient* was sent to two reviewers by my editor and to a third reviewer by me. All found the book worthy of publication; two suggested minor revision, but one of the external referees provided a very lengthy and very constructive critique. The degree to which I make my thesis clear and extricate it from any tendency toward a memoir is a direct result of this referee's critique. This was my intent in writing this book, and I am grateful to the reviewer and the publication process for helping me approach that goal.

UNC Press has been my publishing home for a decade. My long-standing editor, David Perry, retired recently, and Joe Parsons inherited me. The relationship between an author and his editor is a dynamic that is not predictable; I remain very fortunate. Joe has the patience, skills, and sense of humor to help me tell my story. Likewise, the extraordinary longtime director of UNC Press, Kate Douglas Torrey, recently retired. Her successor, John Sherer, has not missed a step. It is an honor to be an author of one of America's premier university presses at a time when it is at the forefront of the transition to this new era of publishing.

By the
Bedside of the
Patient

The Echoing of Medical Humanism

Two generations ago, "physician" was a generic term denoting a medical doctor licensed to practice healing arts. There was specialization, but it was after World War II that subspecialization began in earnest, particularly within the academy. Out in their communities, general practitioners, surgeons, internists, and pediatricians all considered themselves to be physicians and were licensed to practice medicine and surgery in all states. They were all "doctors," professionals who commanded comparable respect regardless of any tendency to restrict their clinical purview. They were considered to be well-educated, highly skilled, and, above all, motivated to do well by their patients. In postwar America, doctors were recourse for the ill.

Today, as specialists are laying claim to particular diseases and body parts, one would be hard-pressed to define "physician." Furthermore, "doctor" denotes a panoply of professionals. Many if not most holding a doctorate have little to do with the healing arts. And within the realm of the healing arts, doctorates abound, as do various licenses designating and sanctioning a range of skills. Some are licensed to perform procedures that overlap with or are identical to those permitted by doctors holding medical licensure, such as Doctors of Osteopathy. Others are licensed for dramatically different practices. Adding to this menu are a great number of caring professionals who are licensed without doctorates—nurses and nurse practitioners, various forms of physician extenders, and all sorts of allied health professionals and sectarian practitioners. Today, recourse for the ill is a far cry from "go to the doctor."

By the Bedside of the Patient is not an exposition on the evolution of doctoring. It takes as its focus one relationship: the sacred trust between the doctor of medicine and the person who chooses to be that doctor's patient. In order to examine the relationship, one needs an appreciation of the roles of the participating doctor and patient and the rules that govern their interaction. None of this is fixed over time or across cultures; what is considered "good" by a constituent in one period may be derided by another in a different place and time. Furthermore, since the end of World War II, the governing rules and the expectations of the participants have changed repeatedly with dizzying speed, never fully predictably or in register.

The medical doctor, the physician, has a role in the contemporary American scene that is far less clear, far less formed, and far less exalted than in most previous eras. More important, the traditional patient-doctor relationship is far less privileged. There are constraints and intrusions that are superimposed by the structure of the contemporary health-care system. Most physicians feel a degree of anxiety beyond that of their forebears as a consequence of these shifting sands, and as a result, many older physicians now choose retirement long before what they foresaw when they entered the profession. They may feel that constraints are imposed on the doctor-patient relationship that go beyond their loss of authority and control in the system; they feel constraints that compromise a well-meaning physician's ability to treat his or her patients to the best of his or her ability, let alone according to conscience. Whether this is a reflection of their own rigidity, a tendency toward being Luddites, or prescience and ethical grounding, the result is stressful. The legendary internist Sir William Osler warned of the dire personal and clinical consequences of a loss of "Aequanimitas"[1] more than a century ago. A physician coping with burdens of this nature is hard-pressed to focus on the needs of the patient, just as the patient coping with illness is confounded by psychosocial challenges in the context in which he is suffering the illness.

These psychosocial challenges are not new, just differently framed. Patients have always had to consider the cost of medical care, but today the consideration goes far beyond their pocketbooks to the tangled worlds of health insurance. For nearly everyone, much is at stake, including the possibility of bankruptcy. Furthermore, patients have to negotiate the administrative maze that exists between them and their doctor. Finally, the rules of the patient-doctor interaction are increasingly difficult to capture with a term such as "satisfaction."

By the Bedside of the Patient focuses on the evolution of the role of the modern physician. Each chapter examines a major post–World War II transition in sequence, dissecting the educational, societal, and policy dialectics at work. Of course, a transition in the role of the physician necessitates a transition in the role of the patient and in the rules of their coming together. *By the Bedside of the Patient* is, thus, an exposition on the dynamics of medical professionalism, the fashion in which professionalism is reframed in response to pressure and preconception brought to bear by the community to be served.

Reductio ad Absurdum

Every adult knows intuitively what "health," "illness," and "doctor" mean. But these words mean something quite different today than they did a decade ago and the decade before that. Articulating definitions is challenging. Health is more than the absence of illness, just as illness is more than the absence of health. But how much more and in what way reflects preconceived notions. Likewise, a "doctor" is no longer a synonym for "medical doctor," and "medical doctor" is often thought of as a collection of technical skills. All these preconceptions are products of culture—the common sense, the comfortable parlance, the relevant institutions, and supporting structures such as marketing, government regulations, and insurance schemes. "Health," "illness," and "doctor" are but three of many core concepts of society that are products of contemporary culture. As is true of all social constructions, they vary from culture to culture in both a geographic sense and a temporal sense. Today's iterations are bolstered by the remarkable reach of technology. Health, illness, and the doctor pop up at all of us all the time on whatever "platform" we engage. Health is a commodity and illness a product line to a degree that was never possible before. And for the "doctor," caring for a patient means walking a tightrope between humanism and consumerism.

The American medical profession of today is a version that bears many more flaws than attributes from its tendency to accumulate the defects rather than the virtues of the iterations that came before. Medical humanism—the desire to bring patient and physician together as people who share the need to define health and seek its nurture—is the attribute that has suffered most in this dialectic. That is not to say that the institution of American medicine is not supporting leaders who proclaim medical humanism almost as a mantra and claim to be marching to its drum. But its pursuit differs from past generations in that the means often have become the end. We are convinced that by doing *something* we have served our patients, and that simply "being there for them" is an antiquated notion not worthy of reimbursement. Medical humanism demands the profession return to the bedside to practice medicine one patient at a time with the highest ethical goals. Health care without an empathic therapeutic relationship might salve disease, but, short of an incisive cure, it does little to salve the suffering inherent in the experience of illness. To serve as a physician requires a concerted and ongoing attempt to define the limits of certainty in a scientific sense and to formulate the boundaries of value in a collaboration that recruits the patient, the patient's community, and the physician's peer group. There is little about this that can be preempted by algorithms or guidelines, and very little that can be delegated to others. Medical humanism demands a doctor-patient relationship that is trustworthy and therapeutic.

However, such a belief may sound hollow and obsolete today. The social constructions of both health and illness have grown reductionistic beyond reason. We are driven to conclusions by metrics that are often obscure, if not irrelevant to the health of the particular patient. For example, when we learn that a particular substance reduces the risk of a particular outcome by some impressive number, say 50 percent, our attention is commanded. But we seldom ask whether we should care. If the reduction reflects a decrease in incidence in the outcome from two in a thousand in a year for those who do not take the substance to one in a thousand for those who do, should we care? And what if the outcome is not that important in terms of our well-being? Are we supposed to care then?

We can impute much more to metrics and numbers that relate to illness and health than humanism supports. Americans walk away from their doctor-patient relationship focused on their body mass index (BMI), serum cholesterol, Hemoglobin A1c, bone mineral density, blood pressure, etc., and both the doctor and the patient consider this a meaningful event. Such metrics are now used to monitor the quality of care despite science that questions their validity. It's as if the Dow Jones Index is a valid window on the health of society and unemployment rates a valid window on the lack thereof. The contemporary social construction of health, illness, and the doctor has fallen victim to what Alfred North Whitehead termed "the fallacy of the misplaced concreteness."[2] It is not that the numbers are irrelevant or that the scientific inferences fallacious; it is that they are incomplete—often sorely incomplete—windows into health and the experience of illness.

There is little likelihood that many of us, even those of us who have acquired the necessary quantitative skills, can sort this out for ourselves when we are ill. We are all inundated with the noise of marketing, the unforgettable anecdote of what happened to another, and the vagaries of clinical science. We are seeking to formulate our values with unreliable measures of benefits and risks knowing that we'd be hard-pressed even if the estimates were reliable.[3] We know from survey data that most often most of us undertake this decision analysis at "home," relying on our common sense and whatever inputs we garner in our community. We choose to be a patient when we lack confidence in this homegrown process. This is the initiation of doctor-patient collaboration in clinical decision making. My goal in writing *By the Bedside of the Patient* is to promote a vision of the role of the "doctor" that is appropriate to the state of the science and the notions of health and illness going forward into the twenty-first century. It is a call for all who aspire to be physicians and all who are in the process of becoming physicians to be disabused of the notion that technical skills, be they in decision theory or surgical methods, are all that is necessary to be a "doctor." The more demanding prerequisite is trustworthiness, the commitment to understand the patient's narrative of illness as comprehensively as one can.

Few events in life render us more vulnerable than when we feel compelled to turn to a fellow human being in quest of wisdom, guidance, empathy, and concern when faced with the experience of illness. Few interactions have the potential to be as intimate. For a physician to do justice to the plea of a patient, to be able to minister to the needs of that particular person, he or she must have a deep understanding of the humanness of the patient's predicament and of the terror and uncertainty that often are hallmarks of that predicament. No patient views an illness as a grand opportunity to engage in an intellectual exercise. To be responsive, the physician must couch the science of medicine in the philosophies of the life experience. Even an obvious idiom of distress, "My wrist hurts because I fell on it," is not so obvious to the patient whose sense of invincibility is threatened. The healing act goes well beyond the diagnosis and setting of a fracture. And when the idiom is far less obvious—such as, "My back is killing me"— the healing act calls for the mobilization of the wisdom of the ages to establish the trust that facilitates understanding of the seemingly counterintuitive scientific basis for therapy.

The doctor-patient relationship includes an understanding of the limitations of certainty regarding challenges in diagnosis and therapy. But that's the easiest part. Seldom is the correct choice obvious. More frequently, there needs to be discussions of options, contingencies, values, and proclivities. If the "correct" choice remains elusive, no patient should ever again ask, "Doc, what would you do?" The question today should be, "Doc, what would you do if you were me?" That question, in this sequence, embodies medical humanism. The grounding in scientifically tested evidence of measured reliability has only become possible in the past fifty years and only grown substantial in the course of the past twenty-five.

The Value of the Human Being

The doctor's role in the doctor-patient relationship has always claimed to be an exercise in humanism. The notion of humanism predates the Renaissance. It is a notion that has a colorful history, with variants that digress into antitheistic, even militant, secularism. I am not inclined to follow that path. For me, humanism is an ideology that espouses reason, ethics, and justice as the pillars of a human-centered philosophy, a philosophy that invokes no agency beyond personal responsibility for one's actions and thoughts. I do not discard or discount religion as contributing to my patient's human nature, her humanity. My patient is a human being who has voiced a predicament that deserves consideration in her own context, however it is framed. The goal of the physician is the well-being of the patient in that relevant context, whether it is a terminal illness, a chaotic home life, or an ecclesiastic calling. The responsibility of the physician is to view the patient's predicament as more than an idiom of distress; it is a window into the way her sense of herself is threatened. The physician's response to that plea is grounded in sheer, uncompromising humanism. Is the patient better off as a consequence of the relationship with the physician, whether the predicament is a terminal illness or a reflection of a recalcitrant adverse psychosocial context?

Likewise, the measure of a "health-care system" is not just its technical prowess and accessibility, or even its clinical outcomes. It is the degree to which it facilitates the social construction of health from a humanist's perspective. Are people better off? That is a measure that is more meaningful than the average blood pressure in the population. The contribution of medicine to attaining the goal of "better off" depends on the degree to which the health-care system promotes trust by the patient for the caregivers and trustworthiness by those involved in the caring. The humanist physician marches to the drumbeat of the needs of the patient, not of the physician or the system.

Of all the iterations of the American health-care system I have lived with, it is the current iteration that does the most to denigrate these tenets. We spend vast fortunes treating type 2 diabetes and other aspects of the "metabolic syndrome" to little if any meaningful avail, but we ignore the disaffection that accompanies social deprivation, which is a far more reproducible assault on both psychological and physiological well-being. And rather than promote and celebrate the trustworthiness of the doctor to help inform medical decisions, we turn to guidelines and algorithms. We have created regulations for the "Electronic Health Record" that demand a "meaningful use" document be handed the patient, as if this is an indication of meaningful care.

By the Bedside of the Patient examines the evolution of what it means to be a doctor over the past sixty years. Sanctioned and applauded attributions of the role of the doctor in one era are replaced by other attributions in the next. Some were discarded none too soon, and some were lost to the detriment of the common good. There are lessons to be had from every transition, which I will provide in later chapters. I have been working in hospitals for all of these sixty years, the last forty-five as a licensed medical doctor. I have witnessed many of these lessons as they played out.

Medical anthropologists would call a book such as this one an "autoethnography." As a clinical investigator trained for rigorous quantification, I am driven to identify sources that corroborate my observations and experiences over this long period. I will provide a paper trail for the sociopolitical and economic constraints I detail decade by decade, a historiography, when such is possible. However, systematic assessments of the practice of medicine lagged behind systematic assessments of medical interventions by decades; the former gained steam only after the Kefauver-Harris Amendment to the federal Food, Drug, and Cosmetic Act, pertaining to pharmaceuticals, was passed in 1962. Most of the literature assessing aspects of the practice of medicine remained anecdotal until the late twentieth century. It is a descriptive literature written by other observers; some of it is a paper trail of my personal perspectives set down in many essays, invited editorials, commentaries, and op-eds I felt compelled to write and publish along the way. I also take advantage of the narratives of my mentors and colleagues, mainly physicians with whom I interacted in the various settings we will examine. Each setting caused me to examine my values, and several required me to make choices. I will display both consequences when they are critical to the ethnography with as much objectivity as I can muster. However, I do not attempt to parse generalizable insights from this anecdotal literature. Hence, the earlier chapters of *By the Bedside of the Patient* are another contribution to an anecdotal literature. I was truly blessed by the mentoring I was afforded and the settings in which I spent the first half of my career as a physician. I unabashedly offer up my anecdotes, as depersonalized as I can make them, in deference to these mentors and these settings. Most were state of the art and state of the science at the time. I have tried to do as well by many students over many decades as the state of the art and the state of the science evolved, and now by the readers of *By the Bedside of the Patient*.

I bring more to this exercise than longevity and persistence. In my career, I have been fortunate to have crossed paths with multiple clinical disciplines and built a research track record that ranges from molecular biology to workplace health and safety. My clinical activities have earned me the assortment of acronyms that accompany my title, each a symbol of peer respect. My research activities have been similarly recognized. And I have a career course in which I have been determined to keep true to myself and to my belief that practicing medicine is a privilege and a ministry. I've marched to this drum, taught to this drum, and lived by its beat. Doing so has angered some, even to the extent that more than one roadblock has been erected and more than one invective hurled. I have managed to soldier on thanks to conviction, to the support of my wife, to the encouragement of students and colleagues, and to the accumulation of credentials and publications than render me hard to ignore, let alone dismiss. I can't expect others to be so fortunate in the face of pushback, which is why I don't consider my life course a role model. At best, it's an object lesson for physicians in the generations that follow.

That is also my intent for *By the Bedside of the Patient*. I have made every effort to walk hand in hand with the reader through halls that may not be so hallowed but were the purview of "doctors" and the setting for doctor-patient relationships. I am aiming for the objectivity of an autoethnography, wherein I describe what I saw, rather than a memoir, wherein I describe what I felt. I am far more comfortable discussing recent decades, when science can bolster that objectivity by virtue of more systematic observations of multiple settings that allow reliably general inferences. I have made every effort to expunge personal responses and personal relationships from the narrative. In the early chapters, my success in doing so is far from complete, but such is the nature of anecdotes. I say this unapologetically. After all, I rely on the memories of some extraordinary physicians to bolster my approach if not my recall, memories of my late friend, Mack Lipkin,[4] and the legendary Lewis Thomas.[5]

Can a Medical Humanist Pray?

The title of this book comes from the second line of "The Morning Prayer of the Physician." It clearly has strong religious overtones, but even the most secular reader should be able to discern an ethic that is ageless and far from metaphysical. It has long resonated much more with me than the Hippocratic Oath, which my generation and those that came before mine often recited at medical school graduations.

THE MORNING PRAYER OF THE PHYSICIAN

O God, let my mind be ever clear and enlightened.
By the bedside of the patient let no alien thought deflect it.
Let everything that experience and scholarship have
taught it be present in it and hinder it not in its tranquil work.
For great and noble are those scientific judgments that serve
the purpose of preserving the health and lives of Thy creatures.

Keep far from me the delusion that I can accomplish all things.
Give me the strength, the will, and the opportunity
to amplify my knowledge more and more.
Today I can disclose things in my knowledge which yesterday
I would not yet have dreamt of, for the Art is great,
but the human mind presses on untiringly.

In the patient let me ever see only the man.
Thou, All-Bountiful One, hast chosen me to watch over
the life and death of Thy creatures.
I prepare myself now for my calling.
Stand Thou by me in this great task, so that it may prosper.
For without Thine aid man prospers not even in the smallest
    things.

The "Morning Prayer" is a legacy of medicine in the caliphates, written around the turn of the last millennium. It has long been debated as to whether to attribute the "Morning Prayer" to Moses Maimonides or to Avicenna. Both were polyglots and polymaths, scholars of great repute and influence. Both were philosophers, theologians, and physicians whose legacy includes great works that influenced Oriental and Western thinking for many generations. Maimonides lived in the twelfth century, Avicenna a century earlier. Assad Meymandi is a contemporary polyglot and polymath who was raised in Persia and earned an M.D. from George Washington University and a Ph.D. in philosophy from the Sorbonne before establishing his practice in psychiatry in North Carolina. He is a musicologist, author, and philanthropist. Doctor Meymandi argues that the attribution belongs to Avicenna.

Neither Avicenna nor Maimonides wrote the prayer presented here, although this version is fully consistent with the teachings of both men. The prayer as we know it first appeared in print in 1793, penned by the German physician Marcus Herz, a student of Immanuel Kant and physician to Moses Mendelssohn. The "Morning Prayer" has had a life of its own, handed down from generation to generation of physicians. Each of its lines is a guidepost for medical practice.

The Legacy of Nineteenth-Century Clinical Humanism

There is a tradition in medicine of the senior physician writing an exhortation for the novitiate, usually offering insights and advice earned during an illustrious career. Many of these essays are cherished to this day by physicians of my generation, casting their long shadows over the likes of *By the Bedside of the Patient.* Fewer and fewer of successive generations of physicians are inclined to seek wisdom in the past. One of these precious essays, Sir William Osler's "Aequanimitas," was mentioned above. Osler considers imperturbability a particularly valuable virtue for the physician who must cope with "the uncertainty which pertains not alone to our science and arts but to the very hopes and fears which make us men." I can attest that equanimity is rarely a feature of the life of the physician in practice today, and it probably never has been.

Osler stands in the clinical pantheon, next to the likes of Maimonides, as a physician who approached the care of the patient as a humanist and who was exquisitely informed by the science of the day. Osler was a Canadian who finished his career at Oxford University but made his mark at the turn of the twentieth century at the newly established Johns Hopkins Medical School in Baltimore. The beginning the last century saw a dramatic watershed in clinical medicine: anesthesia revolutionized surgical possibilities, modern bacteriology was emerging from the miasma, and physiology and biochemistry were casting off metaphysical empiricisms. It was a heady time when American academic medicine became enamored of the reductionism of Prussian science, which put a premium on defining the particular biological causes of disease as if that discovery alone would salve the miseries of mankind. The medical school at Johns Hopkins pioneered this shift in emphasis in the American academy, a shift away from the Cartesian model that had held sway since the American Revolution. Osler's humanism provided balance as medical theory and practice were being transformed at their core.

Harvard Medical School had contributed many to this pantheon of humanist physicians long before the merchant Johns Hopkins endowed his university. Not surprisingly, several of Osler's peers at Harvard shared his devotion to the humanist tradition and the compulsion to champion the perspective with words that will ring true as long as there are ill people and committed clinicians. Francis Weld Peabody was born into a prominent New England family in 1881 and died in 1927, at age forty-six, from sarcoma. After graduating from Harvard Medical School and training at the Massachusetts General Hospital, he sampled medical thinking in Berlin, Peking, and Leningrad in preparation for leaving two indelible marks on Harvard and the world at large: he developed the famous Thorndike Memorial Laboratory and the Harvard teaching service at Boston City Hospital, which produced many a major physician/scientist before it succumbed to Boston's budgetary knife in 1974; and he set a high standard for the teaching of clinical medicine at the bedside and in the lecture hall. As for the latter, he delivered a series of lectures to medical students titled "The Care of the Patient." One lecture, published in the *Journal of the American Medical Association* on March 19, 1927 (volume 88, pages 877–82), is a classic exposition on humanism in medicine. Most who know it remember in particular its last line: "One of the essential qualities of the clinician is interest in humanity, for the secret of the care of the patient is in caring for the patient."

Peabody, as with Osler, welcomed the introduction of reductionistic science into the practice of medicine, a science that probed for the cause of diseased organs as the window on the cause of the diseased patient. He argues that while "absorbed in the difficult task of digesting and correlating new knowledge, it has been easy to overlook the fact that the application of the principles of science to the diagnosis and treatment of disease is only one limited aspect of medical practice [which] includes the whole relationship of the physician with his patient." In other words, "The treatment of a disease may be entirely impersonal; the care of a patient must be completely personal," whether in the office or the dehumanizing milieu of the hospital. With this as his mantra, Peabody was unwilling to treat only those whose illness conformed to the "medical illnesses" that were declared certain and therefore legitimate in that day.

Humanism for the Patient with Symptoms
That Defy Diagnosis

Of the many shortcomings of a reductionistic approach to the care of the patient, few cause more consternation for the patient and for the physician than when no convincing cause for the patient's symptoms can be discerned. Physicians have long been inclined to take the path of least resistance when faced with this conundrum, applying labels to this lack of explanation that range from the theoretical to the fatuous. Anything other than such obfuscating labels might be seen as an admission of the limitations of the physician's competency or a confession about the inadequacy of the state of clinical science. In any case, these labels provide a way to dismiss the patient's concerns without angering him or her or making the physician seem less all-knowing. Peabody, the humanist, was keenly sympathetic to the plight of the patient whose symptoms defied diagnostic acumen. He decried dismissing these patients with, "There really is nothing the matter with you. . . . I'll give you a tonic to take when you go home." Patients with symptoms of unknown origin were a challenge in Peabody's time, just as they are today: "Numerically, then, these patients constitute a large group, and their fees go a long way toward spreading butter on the physician's bread." Peabody argued that dismissing them drives them to try "chiropractic or perhaps . . . Christian Science." Besides, while not being a reassuring diagnosis, "nothing the matter" is also not a tenable concept because, "except for a few low grade morons and some poor wretches who want to get in out of the cold, there are not many people who become hospital patients unless there is something the matter with them. And, by the same token, I doubt whether there are many people except for those stupid creatures who would rather go to the physician than go to the theater, who spend their money on visiting private physicians unless there is something the matter with them."

Peabody expressed great empathy for these patients suffering symptoms of unknown origin. He was uncomfortable with the labels current at a time when psychoanalysis and psychosomatics were in flower, labels such as "psychoneurosis." He felt that since the practice of internal medicine "takes pride in the fact that it concerns itself with the functional capacity of organs rather than with mere structural changes . . . is it not rather narrow minded to limit one's interest to those disturbances of function which are based on anatomic abnormalities?" It follows that the patients with symptoms of unknown origin have "functional disorders," and "the successful diagnosis and treatment of these patients . . . depends almost wholly on the establishment of that intimate personal contact between physician and patient."

James J. Putnam, M.D., was another Brahmin on the Harvard Medical School faculty alongside Peabody. Putnam was the professor of neurology and a pioneer in discerning the pathological processes underlying neurological diseases. However, at the time, the academic disciplines of philosophy, psychology, and neurology had yet to fully differentiate; to this day, the board that certifies competence in neurology also certifies competence in psychiatry. Putnam was drawn to the plight of patients whose symptoms defied pathoanatomical diagnosis. The Shattuck Lecture is an exalted oration named for an eighteenth-century Boston physician and still delivered annually before the Massachusetts Medical Society. Putnam delivered his lecture on June 13, 1899, and it was published in the *Boston Medical and Surgical Journal* (which later became the *New England Journal of Medicine*) the next month (volume 141, pages 53–57). The title is "Not the Disease Only, but Also the Man," and Putnam's focus is the patient whose symptoms defy diagnosis. The jargon of his day included "hysteria" and "psychoneurosis." But notions of "habit diseases" were also bandied about, along with postulates as to their "social etiology." To treat these patients, the physician must "learn . . . to speak and comprehend the mental language of all sorts of conditions of men."

Osler, Peabody, and Putnam are exemplars. They were leading advocates of a scientific basis for modern medicine a century ago. But they knew that science offered only a partial solution for the miseries that drove people to become patients. These legendary clinicians and teachers realized that the experience of illness is always contextual. Hopes and dreams are as susceptible to dissolution and damage as any organ system, or more so; in fact, they can suffer the harmful effects of illness even when organ systems are spared. Society may need practitioners who are skilled in techniques and others who are wedded to advancing technologies, but patients need physicians who are committed to their humanity. Erik Erikson captured this perfectly with a quotation from a patient: "Doctor, my bowels are sluggish, my feet hurt, my heart jumps—and you know, Doctor, I myself don't feel so well either."[6]

Of all the pronouncements and prejudices I heard and the primitive clinical science I witnessed when I started wandering hospital corridors in the 1950s, it was the strains of medical humanism that captured me most. They shaped the content of my undergraduate curriculum and the intensity I brought to the learning. It is my creed as a physician. The first line of the last stanza of the "The Morning Prayer of the Physician" is my creed as a physician and the thesis of this book: "In the patient, let me ever see only the man." I intend to take the reader by the hand and, beginning in the 1950s, travel decade by decade to observe the varying fate of this tenet. There are golden moments, and there are periods of fool's gold. We have begun the twenty-first century in the latter period, with the fate of the tenet and medical professionalism hanging in the balance.

CHAPTER ONE

The Doctor, the Patient, and the
Hospitals of the 1950s

Nothing is distinctive about Parker Street in the southeast Bronx. Many frame houses stand side by side, most now multifamily. There is the occasional shop, and since 2008 there has been a nondescript eight-story apartment house at 1424. The Parker Street neighborhood is part of an area called "Parkchester" because it abuts the apartment complex of that name, one of several remarkable experiments in urban planning undertaken by the Metropolitan Life Insurance Company in the aftermath of World War II.

MetLife traces its roots to the time of the Civil War. It grew to be a dominant force in its industry early in the twentieth century. Many aspects of this industry have an "actuarial" business model, which means that they adjust premiums to cover potential payouts going forward. The consequence, often, is the accumulation of enormous financial war chests and a propensity to invest heavily in whatever seems likely to be lucrative. The crash of the stock market in 1929 cost MetLife dearly and caused its leadership to seek alternative investments. In 1932 they lobbied aggressively and successfully for the repeal of legislation that barred insurance companies from investing in real estate. Rather than solely purchase existing investment properties, however, MetLife's leadership opted to create neighborhoods that could be afforded by families with modest incomes. Parkchester was one such neighborhood. MetLife purchased 129 acres of farmland from the Catholic Protectorate; the Catholic home for troubled boys on that property was moved to Westchester County. Between 1939 and 1942, 171 apartment buildings were constructed at a cost of $50 million. The buildings were eight- and twelve-story brick structures with lots of patios. Strikingly, they were not arrayed on a grid; they were built around a central "oval" and separated as on a campus with green spaces and recreational facilities. Automobile access was limited to two main roads. Parkchester was very successful in attracting upwardly mobile families, including those headed by returning veterans after the end of World War II. The result was a very dynamic multiethnic, albeit racially segregated, community. Retail establishments dotted the two main roads. There were no clinics or hospitals.

That brings us back to 1424 Parker Street. From 1929 until it closed in March 1978, this was the site of Parkchester General Hospital. It was a 178-bed general hospital until 1959, when a four-story wing was added, increasing the bed count to 208. The wing and other renovations were in response to a threat from the New York State Hospital Commission to deny Parkchester licensure unless it was brought up to the newly enacted hospital codes. The daily room charge was a substantial out-of-pocket sum for most families, few of whom had any sort of health or hospital insurance. Many physicians, usually general practitioners in the Bronx, were invited to admit their patients to this hospital; my father was one of them. I was employed by the hospital on weekends and summers from about 1955 to 1960. My tasks ranged from drawing bloods to working in the clinical laboratory and serving as a "circulating nurse" (a step-and-fetch) in the operating rooms. I became immersed in its culture.

Parkchester General Hospital was a proprietary hospital, privately owned and operated for profit. About 15 percent of the hospitals across postwar America were proprietary, most owned by a physician or group of physicians. There are descriptive statistics[1] and policy statements for these hospitals. For example, New York City mayor Robert Wagner appointed a Commission on Health Services that conducted a seventeen-month survey and advised "a broad reorganization of the city's health and hospital services."[2] The report called for the affiliation of municipal hospitals with medical schools and/or voluntary teaching hospitals. It also called for "closer supervision by the city of proprietary hospitals" and a discontinuance of the "licensing of unaccredited proprietary hospitals." The commission decried the employment of untrained and poorly trained personnel in clinically responsible roles. Clearly, a sea change was under way in the 1960s in New York City and across the nation.

But very little was published about the experience of the doctor or the patient in these proprietary hospitals before the sea change started, particularly anything that was derived from systematic studies. That is a much more recent undertaking and the focus of the later chapters in this book. Hence, there is no way to know if Parkchester General Hospital was representative in this regard, but even if it is an outlier, it certainly is a telling outlier. For many working-class patients, these proprietary hospitals offered a degree of comfort, convenience, and privacy that was more appealing than the ambience of publicly funded hospitals and more affordable than "voluntary" hospitals underwritten by philanthropists or established by various religious orders. Proprietary hospitals also appealed to private physicians, many of whom did not have admitting privileges to the not-for-profit voluntary hospitals. The proprietary hospitals welcomed their business and allowed them to commandeer their patients' hospital course and their fee-for-service remuneration.

Parkchester General Hospital was owned by Charles L. Engelsher, M.D. Dr. Engelsher graduated from the New York University Medical School in 1925 and pursued a career as a general surgeon. Neither formal residency training nor board certification was prerequisite to being a general surgeon in his day—only loose apprenticeship, practice, and hubris were requisites. The American Board of Surgery was not founded until 1937. For that matter, in most states, any licensed M.D. or Doctor of Osteopathy can perform surgery today if offered access to an appropriate venue. Engelsher apparently managed quite a profitable practice, so profitable that he purchased Parkchester General Hospital in 1940. A clue to his financial success can be found in testimonies before a Moreland Act commission in 1943. The Moreland Act was passed by the New York legislature in 1907 to empower the governor to appoint a commission "to investigate the management and affairs of any department, board, bureau or commission of the state." In 1943 the commission was looking into irregularities of the administration of the workmen's (today termed workers') compensation scheme in the Bronx. There are colorful reports in the *Yonkers Herald Statesman* (June 11, 1943) and *Mount Vernon Daily Argus* (June 12, 1943) about the relationships between Joseph "Socks" Lanza (a convicted "fish market racketeer"), Zangwill Engelsher (Charles's brother), and union officers that resulted in workmen's compensation cases being directed to Parkchester General Hospital. If not a racketeer himself, Charles Engelsher was quite a raconteur. He was described as a "willing and jovial witness" in workmen's compensation trials and was proud of the fact that in the 1940s, a man with a criminal record had "more of a chance of getting a job with me than if he had led a blameless life." He denied impropriety, but when asked if Parkchester General Hospital was more of a reform school than a hospital, he said, "It's a little of both."

By the time I knew the hospital and the good doctor, both had assumed the mantle of respectability that follows from Engelsher's heavy personal and financial involvement in Democratic politics in the Bronx. He even enjoyed his fifteen minutes of fame, which doubtless would have been far longer if the episode happened in today's media environment. In the summer of 1957, he rushed to the site of a horrific crash of a train on a nearby elevated platform. The lead car dangled over the pavement for hours while firefighters tried to free the motor-man pinned inside—unsuccessfully, until Engelsher amputated his leg. Engelsher died at home in 1964 at age sixty-two. His obituary in the *New York Times* on August 26, 1964, does not pull many punches regarding the good doctor's various political shenanigans.

The Parkchester General Hospital I knew was a monument to Engelsher's imperiousness. He was driven to the front door in a pink Cadillac and fawned upon by the staff as he passed through his domain. He led an entourage to the bedsides of his patients, anointing some with a rose (literally), and all with a benediction. The top floor had been converted into his penthouse, where he lived much of the workweek and entertained often, leaving many a ribald tale as witness. He returned to his Long Island estate on the weekends, the site of the semiannual wining and dining of the physicians who admitted patients to his fiefdom. If there were still convicts on staff, I was unaware. But the nepotism was blatant, from siblings to Engelsher's brother-in-law, a mild-mannered "surgeon" who had gone offshore for his medical degree.

Charles Engelsher was in his greatest glory in the operating rooms. The operating "theater" of the 1950s was a far cry from that of today. Regulations were nearly nonexistent. The technology to deliver anes-thetics in a tightly monitored fashion through tubes inserted into the trachea had not been developed. Ether was still dripped on a face mask while the patient was manually restrained to keep him or her safe through the phase of agitation that preceded the unconsciousness that allowed surgery to proceed. (Ether had been used as a party drug for decades before its anesthetic properties were demonstrated; apparently, "ether frolics" offered something desirable.) Many of the procedures that were the bread and butter of proprietary hospitals in the 1950s have long fallen out of favor, some even before they were scrutinized through scientific testing. Tonsillectomies and radical mastectomies met this fate, only to be replaced subsequently by many other procedures, several of which are still in common practice despite a lack of scientific evidence of their efficacy, or even evidence from nonscientific sources.

The clinical laboratory was a small room staffed by a couple of trained technologists. They drew blood from patients and analyzed blood and urine for the limited assortment of tests that were available at that time. In the 1950s, blood glucoses was still determined by the multistep Folin-Wu method developed at Harvard in the 1920s, and blood counts were determined by counting cells under the microscope. All of this was done by hand; today, it is automated with analytical machines capable of myriad tests on an enormous number of samples.

My mentor at Parkchester General Hospital was Dr. Julius Cohen. Julie was a graduate of Middlesex Medical School, which taught "eclectic medicine," one of the alternatives to my medical profession that came into existence in the nineteenth century. In 1928 Middlesex Medical School moved into what is now the "Castle" in the middle of the Brandeis University campus in Waltham, Massachusetts. It had a faculty of some forty physicians, all licensed as medical doctors and nearly all experienced generalists. According to its bulletin, it offered a premedical curriculum and a medical curriculum that was standard and comprehensive for its day (http://archive.org/details/bulletin192930midd).

Many sectarian healing movements came into existence in nineteenth-century America, and several are still in existence today, including chiropractic, osteopathy, the Pentecostal Movement, Christian Science, and naturopathy, to name a few. "Eclectic medicine" did not survive the antipathy of the American Medical Association. Eclectic medicine viewed my chosen guild, termed "allopathic" medicine by the homeopaths, as yet another form of a "sect" that maintained a rigid set of beliefs and practices sanctioned by its "seniors" who dismissed all other belief systems. The Middlesex bulletin quotes Dr. John King, a proponent of eclectic medicine, who stated in 1870 that "the liberal and humane spirit of the age is opposed to such intolerance [by the medical mainstream], and demands that sectarians in theology and science shall extend mutual toleration to each other. Such is the kindly and harmonious spirit which American eclectics desire to see introduced into the profession; but in addition to these ethical improvements, they desire a more faithful and prompt adherence to the dictates of CLINICAL EXPERIENCE" (emphasis in the original). The entire bulletin makes for interesting reading. It defends the Middlesex Medical School with a language that is nearly identical to that which promoted the development of rural medical schools across America and elsewhere fifty years later: it emphasizes practice, primary care in rural communities, clinical education and the clinical relevance of classroom teaching, recruiting students from a broader socioeconomic background, recruiting clinical teachers, and the wisdom gained in the course of clinical practice. In terms of the details of the preclinical curriculum, Middlesex differed little from Harvard, a powerful and self-congratulatory beacon situated some twenty miles downstream on the Charles River. But Middlesex Medical School did not aspire to be elite, or to have a presence in the research community, or to build a citadel. After all, it was 1929, and medical science was a stirring phoenix yet to emerge from the ashes of dogmatism. Aside from opiates, very little in the allopathic pharmacopoeia offered the possibility of benefit, and much was harmful. Surgery was also in its infancy and not represented in the graduate curriculum; it was sampled by interns in the requisite postgraduate year in a hospital, a year required for the licensure of Middlesex graduates as well as allopathic graduates. As best I can tell, Middlesex Medical School was fifty years ahead of its time.

At the turn of the century, America was dotted with all sorts of schools of the "healing arts." In 1910 the educator Abraham Flexner published the results of a survey sponsored by the Carnegie Foundation of the number and quality of these institutions. By 1929, only sixty-one of the 121 "allopathic" medical schools that had been operating in 1901 remained open. Most that closed were "storefront" operations, far less structured than Middlesex Medical School, but the Flexnerian sweep also took out the medical schools affiliated with Dartmouth and Bowdoin Colleges. Of twenty-two homeopathic schools, only two remained, and only two of twelve eclectic schools remained: Middlesex and the Eclectic Medical College of Cincinnati, which already had announced its closing. The American Medical Association declared that Middlesex was not a medical school, but it hung on for a short while longer by the grace of the Massachusetts legislature. By the time Julie Cohen graduated in 1932, no state recognized his degree as a credential for licensure.

After graduating from Middlesex, Julie took a job as the full-time house physician at Parkchester General Hospital; today, he would be called a "hospitalist." I knew little of his personal life except his pride in his son, "Brucie," who was a student at Yale Law School. Julie knew the occupants of the hospital beds not just by their location and diagnosis but through conversations with them. All the patients had a private physician, often Charles Engelsher. Like Engelsher, many of the other private physicians were present at their patients' bedsides during their occasional rounds. But it was Julie who demonstrated compassion for these patients; he knew who was alone and afraid and who was taking a turn for the worse. Julie taught me that a hospital is either a community of caring people or a terrible place. He valued the nursing staff, the dietary staff, the custodial staff, and all else who worked for the benefit of the patient. These people had names and smiles. They were not reporting to supervisors in separate administrative domains; they had a job to do and appreciated a thank you for a job well done from the likes of a Julie Cohen, who stood with them at the bedside. Of course, I was a kid and in no position to appreciate Julie Cohen's clinical acumen, or lack thereof, beyond bedside manner. I even suspect that his title of "Doctor" was an honorific bestowed by the staff in view of his Middlesex degree rather than a symbol of licensure. After all, as the Wagner Commission had documented, many in clinical roles in inpatient facilities, particularly proprietary and municipal inpatient facilities, were lacking in training, credentials, and licensure.

Much of the treatment of the hospitalized patient in the 1950s began with bed rest. The "rest cure" was the legacy of Silas Weir Mitchell, a Philadelphia physician who popularized it in Victorian times, mainly for women with depression, particularly postpartum depression. However, it has a history that dates to Hippocrates. Bed rest came to dominate medical thinking by the 1950s and has been brought to heel only in the past few decades. Prolonged bed rest was the treatment for rheumatoid arthritis, backache, heart failure, heart attacks, recovery from surgery, and complications of pregnancy and recovery postpartum. Harvard's famous obstetrical hospital was named Boston Lying-In in deference to linguistic determinism, not clinical prescience. Patients in the beds of Parkchester General Hospital were there for prolonged periods. The national average length of stay in "short-term general hospitals rose to 7.8 days in 1959," according to the American Hospital Association survey cited above. An institution such as Parkchester General Hospital became an extension of the homes of many residents of the Parkchester neighborhood, an extension for various spells in their lives from birth till death.

The "bed rest cure" is no longer a defensible prescription. In nearly all clinical settings, there have been systematic scientific studies demonstrating an unfavorable risk/benefit ratio. But that's not the lesson I carried away from rounds with Julie Cohen. The patients in the beds of any hospital are not born to be patients; they are people, nearly all of whom would choose to be participating in their life course without hospitalization. They all need to be made to feel like people, valued individuals as much "at home" as possible until they are at home. Julie and the staff he worked with modeled that behavior. That is ever more challenging today, when inpatient care is horrifyingly fragmented, "care" is often a euphemism for technology, reimbursement favors early discharge, those providing the care report to individuals distant from the bedside, and fewer and fewer of these "caregivers" ever feel the satisfaction of witnessing a sigh of relief or a smile. Julie Cohen may have had limited credentials, but he had no limit to his humanism.

Goldwater Memorial Hospital

I was too young to understand notions of "quality of care" and medical expertise during my Parkchester General Hospital years. Neither my father nor Julius Cohen would praise Parkchester General Hospital in that context. Their esteem was reserved for the prominent, medical school–affiliated hospitals, the hospitals the Wagner Commission wanted to use as regional standards for the development of hospitals in New York City. I knew not why until my senior year in high school. I was nominated for and accepted into the Ford Foundation's legendary Science Honors Program at Columbia University.

The Science Honors Program introduced us to high-quality didactics and an approach to laboratory science. I was also introduced to clinical excellence over lunch one day. Part of the program was a luncheon in the faculty club with Columbia luminaries. One Saturday, I found myself across the table from Beatrice Carrier Seegal. She was professor of microbiology at the medical school, a renowned pioneering immunologist, and a graduate of Johns Hopkins Medical School. I was smitten. She looked like Katharine Hepburn; exuded patience, confidence, and competence; and cared about students. I worked that summer in her laboratory and took my passion for science and scholarship up another notch. But that's not all she did for me. She introduced me to her husband, David Seegal.

David Seegal was a legendary professor of medicine and chief of the Columbia medical service at Goldwater Memorial Hospital on the southern tip of Welfare Island (now called Roosevelt Island) in the middle of the East River. David was a presence, a large personality who enjoyed asking probing questions. Furthermore, he was a legendary bedside teacher; students from Columbia and around the country took elective months at Goldwater just to learn at the feet of the great man. In 1970 the Seegals endowed the "Leaders in Medicine" archive of Alpha Omega Alpha, the medical honorary society. This is a video archive of interviews of many American medical luminaries, starting with a remarkable interview of David Seegal.

Goldwater Memorial Hospital has several claims to everlasting fame. During World War II, the basement of its Building D housed a laboratory developing the antimalarial treatments that were necessary for the war effort in the South Pacific. The young physician-scientists working on this project would go on to make some of the greatest scientific advances of the postwar era. The list includes James Shannon, who developed and directed the modern National Institutes of Health; the pioneering kidney physiologist Robert Berliner; and Jules Axelrod, who would win a Nobel Prize. But this laboratory was a footnote in the

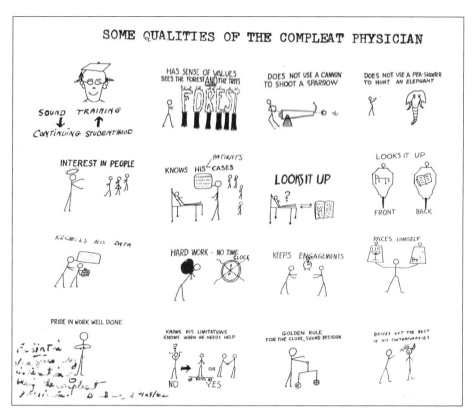

FIGURE 1 David Seegal, "Some Qualities of the Compleat Physician."

Goldwater history. The hospital opened in 1939 as America's first public hospital devoted to the care and study of patients with chronic diseases, and Dr. Seegal moved over from Columbia's Presbyterian Hospital to become director of the Columbia Research Service at Goldwater.

I met with David and Beatrice Seegal on many, many precious occasions. Whenever I returned to New York City on college vacations and later on medical school vacations, I was invited to spend an afternoon with them in their Claremont Avenue apartment in the middle of the Columbia campus. There, David "interviewed" me ceaselessly, often handing me one of his own papers to read aloud and then asking for my interpretation. David would take me on rounds with him on the Goldwater service, an unforgettable experience of witnessing exquisite clinical skills and acumen in the service of compassion and empathy. David knew how to elicit a patient's narrative of illness and demonstrated the art of listening. No doubt my empathy for patients with chronic diseases took root in his shadow and accounts for my career as a rheumatologist.

David Seegal was also a prototype for the great postwar physician,[3] in the tradition of Osler, Peabody, and Putnam discussed in the introduction. He was intensely interested and curious about the illness of every inpatient he saw at Goldwater. He excelled at demonstrating the arts of listening to the narrative of illness and of discerning the physical manifestations of the underlying disease. He mastered the literature of the day that related to the causes of the diseases and the science that pointed the way to the future. But his scholarship ranged far beyond the science that was obviously relevant; he read widely and peppered the medical literature with philosophical essays and poetry, including a desire to put a Western veneer on haiku. He was the exemplar of the humanist physician of his generation and modeled that behavior for all who attended his rounds. I did not realize the chinks in his stately armor until much later. He also modeled imperiousness—not the puffed-up imperiousness of Engelsher at Parkchester, but a consummate paternalism and studied showmanship. This was expected of great physicians of that time. Today, it belongs in the archives of medicine and not at the bedside. Imperiousness aside, David Seegal embodied the drive toward excellence, toward being the "compleat physician."

During an afternoon visit in the spring of my sophomore year in college, David provided me with a photograph, a composite of the slides he had used to deliver an address to an entering medical school class. That photograph is reproduced as figure 1 and is worth a thousand words. David Seegal and Goldwater provided the balance to Parkchester General Hospital that I needed to see medicine's moral high ground and to start the climb.

In 1996 Goldwater Hospital merged with Coler Hospital as a 2,000-bed specialty hospital and nursing facility for the chronically ill. It will soon be a memory, perhaps marked by a monument if the Roosevelt Island Historical Society succeeds in establishing a park on the site. Goldwater-Coler is scheduled for demolition to make way for a high-tech science campus run jointly by Cornell University and the Technion-Israel Institute of Technology. The shadows of its remarkable past will always be present on Roosevelt Island. Maybe the doctors that will come to work and live on this little island in the middle of the East River will be able to see these shadows.

Morrisania Hospital

In colonial times, the land that is now the Bronx, Westchester County, and much of New Jersey was owned by the Morris family. Lewis Morris signed the Declaration of Independence, and Gouverneur Morris penned the Constitution. For generations, a section of what is now the South Bronx was called Morrisania. If Lewis Morris had had his way, it would be the capital of the country. Instead, it remained agrarian until the early twentieth century, when the "elevated railroad" and the subway were extended north from Manhattan—just in time to accommodate the influx of European immigrants. By 1929, the Bronx was Yankee Stadium surrounded by a forest of five- and six-story apartment buildings teaming with immigrants.

Health care of this largely working-class population was a challenge not easily met in a country that was wedded to a fee-for-service model. Jimmy Walker became mayor of New York City in 1926, a time when the economy was robust and the coffers of the city brimming—which Walker's cohorts in Tammany Hall knew all too well. The speakeasies and scandals have been romanticized in many a book and film. Less remembered is the proliferation of public works projects, including the construction of the city's third municipal hospital, Morrisania Hospital. Hizzoner opened the hospital in 1929, declaring, "This institution is a monument to an idea. To public service, and to posterity, I dedicate these buildings."[4]

Morrisania Hospital was a large complex. The main building was the 400-bed hospital and clinic with an ornately decorated façade and distinctive red roof. Of the three other buildings in the complex, two were residences for nurses and other employees and the other was for utilities and laundry. Medical care was provided mainly by volunteering physicians. Morrisania rapidly took its place at the forefront of the development of the twentieth-century municipal hospital system in America's burgeoning cities.[5]

The era between the wars brought transition for American health care. The wealthier citizenry was starting to consider hospitalization a reasonable alternative to home care, and elite physicians were more than happy to see the demands of house calls brought to heel. Hospitals, whether supported by philanthropy or municipal coffers, were walking financial tightropes and started to provide facilities that would compete for the trade. This all came to a screeching halt with the Great Depression. Private, paying patients became a scarcity. The municipal hospitals took on an ever-increasing load and acquired ever-increasing influence despite the restrictions imposed by financial exigencies. Free care was offered only to the needy, but over half the population of New York City qualified.[6]

Municipal hospitals emerged from the war years as thriving and vital institutions, long on patients and staffing needs but short on funds and frills. That did not last long. Jobs, people, and their physicians were rapidly heading to the suburbs, leaving behind little advocacy for these aging facilities. Those who did not leave but could afford care chose private hospitals, including proprietary hospitals such as Parkchester General. The municipal hospitals rapidly slipped into disarray in terms of their facilities and their function, as the report of the Wagner Commission emphasized. In 1961 a Columbia medical professor, Ray Trussel, was appointed commissioner of hospitals with a mandate to do something about the state of the city's municipal institutions. His solution was to develop contractual relationships with private institutions, delegating control and staffing to the latter. Morrisania came under the wing of Montefiore Hospital, an affiliate of the Albert Einstein School of Medicine, but not for long. With the advent of Medicaid and Medicare, much of the patient population desired and were desired by private and not-for-profit hospitals, leaving the aged, hulking municipal facilities relatively unoccupied. Some were refurbished. Some, including Morrisania, were closed.

My father was a GP (general practitioner) in the Bronx who served as a physician in the Morrisania eye clinic for years, initially volunteering and later accepting a token stipend. That he was not a specialist had no bearing on staffing. I often accompanied him to this clinic. I wish I could tell you that facilities like this are no longer to be found in America, but there are many that come close, such as Chicago's Cook County Hospital and Atlanta's Grady Memorial. Rows of benches filling a large room were occupied by minions, all waiting, patiently and submissively, for their names to be called. There followed a brief check-in, an expeditious eye examination, and a prescription for glasses, eye drops, or referral to an ophthalmologist. It's a far cry from the elegance of private optician, optometrist, or ophthalmologist offices, with their comfortable waiting rooms and displays of designer eyeglass frames. However, much of the screening at such places requires no more than could be provided in a Morrisania clinic by an anonymous doctor. And the U.S. military and the British National Health Service discovered long ago that "designer eyeglasses" served nothing more than a marketing agenda; a limited number of functional and understated options served the patients' clinical needs just as well. Even prescription lenses are no longer produced by skilled grinders; they are manufactured in bulk in all ranges of refractive index and often sold at an enormous profit margin. Morrisania and its clinics are gone, but their model for efficiency in terms of "through put" is not. This is the model for many a modern "clinic," except for the cost-effectiveness notion, which is trumped by profitability.

The City Doctor in the 1950s

Charlie Engelsher and David Seegal seemingly had little in common. Engelsher was a medical entrepreneur with local clout, Seegal a prototypical professor with national renown. However, these men had much more in common than is apparent at first blush. Both had overcome considerable political challenges—one in the smoke-filled rooms populated by pols, the other within the more insidious intrigues that have always infested the academy. Both strutted, larger than life, as masters of their fiefdoms. And while both could serve the clinical demands of their patients with the skills they had honed, neither felt compelled to know more than was necessary about the essential humanity of their patients.

Even for David Seegal, whom I hold in the highest regard as a clinical educator for many and a mentor for me, "interest in people" is the sole people-centered element he professed in figure 1—not even "interest in a person" or "interest in a patient," except as it was relevant to his or her disease state. Missing from figure 1 is a dollop of Julie Cohen, who was neither an entrepreneur nor a professor, just a caring man who happened to be a doctor who was unable to get a license to practice his very personal brand of caring in the community.

The challenge for the profession today is to balance these three roles in its membership. The challenge for the physician is to balance these three roles in his or her worldview. The challenge for society is to realize its role in the balancing. What is to be valued, and to what degree? In the 1950s, very few people understood that there was such dialectic, but there were some.

The Tavistock Clinic was founded in London shortly after World War I and gained fame for the treatment of the psychological disorders suffered by veterans of that war. It evolved to be a center of Freudian psychoanalytic thinking and therapy by the time it was to serve veterans of World War II. Many luminaries of psychiatry have served on its staff or passed through its training programs. One of the former was Michael Balint, M.D., Ph.D. Balint was a refugee from Budapest who had been driven to Britain by the advent of Nazi persecution. He is best known in psychoanalytic circles for his writings on the mother-child relationship, but I was introduced to Balint's ideas concerning another subject by Dr. Fred Schactman, a psychologist retired from the staff of the Menninger Clinic. Dr. Schactman was in the audience one night when I was lecturing on the role of the physician in medicalization, and afterward he directed me to a paper by Balint published in *The Lancet* in 1955 and titled "The Doctor, His Patient, and the Illness." This is a remarkable discourse for many reasons, including the fact that neither *The Lancet* nor any other general medical journal is wont to publish a six-page transcript of an address on any clinical topic any longer, let alone the Presidential Address to the British Psychological Association.[7]

In the paper, Balint describes research seminars organized for general practitioners at the Tavistock Clinic that probed the upsides and downsides of "the most frequently used drug in general practice . . . the doctor himself." His thesis is the midcentury version of the arguments offered earlier by Peabody, Osler, and Putnam. He acknowledges that the art of patient care goes well beyond simply caring for the patient. He realizes that in order to initiate medical care, the patient often attempts to "offer or propose a variety of illnesses to the doctor," reflecting the "unstructured" fashion of becoming ill. In response, the physician brings an "apostolic function" to the interview, confronting the "unstructured" illness with preconceptions that reflect training, prejudices, projections, and more. This interaction can structure the illness, determine the quality of the relationship between the doctor and the patient, and inform the doctor's preconceptions going forward. It is a not an interview; it is a dialectic.

Of course, Balint brings his own "apostolic function" to this discussion. He is convinced that this dialectic is cemented in primary care in the first interview between the patient and the general practitioner. He feels the die is long cast by the time a specialist gets involved. He is also convinced that psychodynamics of the interactions are prejudiced by the training of the GP, which is long on biologic diagnoses and therapeutics and short on the painstaking methods of psychoanalysis. We will come to understand in chapters that follow that the dialectic is ongoing throughout the course of illness and across multiple treatment acts and environments. Furthermore, it can be couched in terms that are far less Freudian—as in the 1970s by the likes of Arthur Kleinman, a psychiatrist turned pioneering medical anthropologist. Kleinman's early books defined the notion of symbolic reality in medicine, the need to parse and comprehend the idioms of distress in the narrative the patient constructs to define his illness.[8] The interplay between the patient's need to structure his illness in his terms and the doctor's "apostolic function" plays out within the constraints of culture.[9] Caring for the patient and caring about the patient is a life pursuit for which reductionism, system design, and technology will never be more than infrastructure.

Proprietary hospitals would largely disappear in the 1970s. Regulations as to space per bed, staffing, and much more did violence to their business model. Besides, public and not-for-profit institutions were growing in visibility, size, and scope and were more than willing to appeal to the growing numbers of workers who were provided health insurance by their employers. Interestingly, proprietary hospitals are making a considerable comeback in the twenty-first century, offering enhancements in convenience and ambience—and being willing to expand the scope of the "free" market. They always have a specialty or subspecialty hook: orthopedic hospitals, cardiac hospitals, hospitals specializing in workers' compensation claimants, eye hospitals, and more. They thrive on providing the most lucrative of technological interventions. Most are run by one or a few New Age Charlie Engelshers. I'll have more to say about that in later chapters.

CHAPTER TWO

Academics and Medicine
in the 1960s

The collegiate "liberal arts" tradition is peculiarly American and currently under siege. I found myself defending it while still an undergraduate. David Seegal forced my hand. The Seegals had no children
but had a long track record of identifying students, usually medical
students, of promise as physicians and physician-scientists and nurturing their careers. I may have been the youngest and also the last so
honored by their interest. David Seegal was a broadly educated scholar
with wide-ranging interests, but he was even more the larger-than-life
humanist physician. That was his ambition for me. He did not want
me to remain in the world of arts and sciences without giving medicine a chance to be my life's work. He had no reason for that concern;
medicine was imprinted on me at birth by an immigrant father who
graduated from Harvard Medical School in 1929, pursued a career
in general practice, and wanted a son to return to Harvard Medical
School with the mandate to pursue a career in academic medicine.
I was that son. But David Seegal was sufficiently concerned about my
"calling" that he recruited Louis Lasagna, the pioneering Johns Hopkins pharmacologist, to urge me to apply for early admission to medical school. Despite his entreaties, I would not abbreviate my liberal
arts education. I have always been thankful I made that choice. I am
an unwavering advocate for approaching medicine as a philosophy, a
system of thinking informed by science but not itself a science. And
I am no less an advocate for approaching all walks of life as a moral
philosopher might walk—with awareness, curiosity, skepticism, and
concern. The liberal arts experience promises preparation for such a
walk for any who find it as appealing as I did. Science is but one of the

bodies of information one needs to absorb in order to be prepared to participate in the care of the ill. Medical school curricula have only recently begun to come to this realization, and still very tentatively. Our society will suffer sorely if we yield to those who do not appreciate the virtues of a liberal arts education. I'll return to this argument when we confront the current movement to abbreviate medical education.

Science in college is not a "prerequisite" for medical school, nor is the "premed" designation essential to matriculation toward competence as a physician. Science in college is another rich exposure to rationalism and empiricism worthy of immersion. It is more important to understand the thinking and perspective that drives the academic chemist than it is to get a good grade in "organic chemistry." Yale taught me what scholarship means, what science demands,[1] and what the quest to be an educated person entails. "Premedical" education is the preparation for understanding the eloquence of Avicenna, Rambam, Osler, Peabody, and Putnam, revealed in the introduction, and of others who followed them. It is not an exercise in gaining access to medical school.

Finding "Education" in the Medical School Curriculum: An Odyssey

There is no universal medical school curriculum; there are curricula that are always being targeted for reform by each generation of medical educators. What are less targeted since early in the twentieth century are the overall templates. For European countries and most of their former colonies, students enter medical school after a secondary school education that entails more years than are required for most that enter an undergraduate course of study in the United States. The European medical school curriculum is structured over six years, during which preclinical courses include material that most American medical students are exposed to as undergraduates. The American model includes a four-year undergraduate curriculum with "premedical" requirements in the sciences followed by four years of medical school. How the American version came about is debatable. It appears that much of the medical curriculum has its roots in the University of Edinburgh, which has had a very influential and innovative medical faculty since its founding in the eighteenth century. The Edinburgh faculty developed a curriculum that emphasized all sciences for two years, followed by clinical teaching for another two to three years. This model was copied by Canadian medical schools and adopted by Johns Hopkins Medical School when it opened in Baltimore in 1890. Abraham Flexner took notice.

Ever since the Flexner report, American medical education has entailed two years of didactic teaching and two years of clinical "rotations" or "clerkships." The "preclinical years" are designed to provide the student with the basic scientific knowledge that is considered necessary for all physicians to master. The clinical years are designed to expose the student to the daily work and mindset of clinicians in various specialties and subspecialties. No doubt this paradigm served to expunge some of the shoddiness that characterized nineteenth-century professional education.[2] No doubt it is considered inviolate since only minor tweaking has occurred in some schools over the past century in the United States. Yet there is also no doubt that it is little more than a pedagogically flawed gauntlet.

The obvious pedagogical flaws of the American paradigm relate to the quantity of information presented in the preclinical curriculum and the superficiality of many of the exposures to practice during the clinical years. But neither of these flaws should be a challenge for most medical students. Swallowing great gobs of information is work, but not particularly difficult or stressful work for the kind of candidates that are selected by American medical schools. You just sit down and do it. Much of it is even interesting. Texts are often well written, lecturers often competent, and laboratory exercises mentored by enthusiastic faculty. "Good" medical students quickly learn what is expected of them on each clinical rotation and accept direction with deference if not adulation. Medical school admission committees are primed to find such "good students" in the applicant pool. Four years later, one is comfortable with the language of medicine, its rituals, and its processes. Four years later, one is expected to move on into training for whatever clinical discipline seemed most appealing for whatever reason.

The less-obvious pedagogical flaws relate to whether these exposures during medical school create a clinician who will remain informed in the future or are simply gauntlets to postgraduate education. During the early decades of my career on the faculty of the School

Academics and Medicine in the 1960s

of Medicine at UNC, I was part of the team teaching basic immunology to the first-year class and the musculoskeletal sciences course to the second-year class. I enjoyed teaching these courses; my colleagues were excellent scientists, some clinician-scientists, who took on the task with enthusiasm. The eager though anxious students were a delight to work with. But . . . these preclinical courses generally last about a month and are extremely intense, both in terms of the volume of material and hours in the lecture hall and teaching laboratory. As I mentioned, most of our highly selected students mastered what was expected of them with facility, those with science backgrounds in particular. After each course, the faculty would meet to consider how we might improve the course next year. Each year, I would point out that I see these same students in their third or fourth years when they are immersed in their clinical rotations; their recall of the preclinical content is marginal and not necessary for the daily tasks of the rotations. Many of my colleagues responded that they were teaching to the occasional student whose interest in the material would lead to a career in that particular basic science. I would argue that we need to educate physicians first; the scientist in the herd would find a different pasture. I would further argue that we need a curriculum that builds over time, not one that is so discontinuous. Education in medical school should be viewed as a foundation for Continuing Medical Education throughout the life of the physician. Basic sciences must be taught so as to remain prerequisite to competence regardless of the degree to which graduates restrict their clinical purview in the future. Likewise, the clinical exposures must provide an approach that considers the patient as a human being; no clinician should be applauded for mastery of a part of a person in isolation. Physicians are scholars of the human predicament, or they are not physicians.[3] We have diced and sliced the education of the physician so that the profession is balkanized. Few in practice can do much more than provide lip service to clinical challenges outside their honed purview, most cannot even muster lip service, and many could care not less about their insularity.

The flaws in a staccato and disconnected preclinical curriculum were long obvious and did not escape the attention of my class at Harvard Medical School. We delivered a manifesto to Dean Robert Ebert in the second year. In the 1960s, the dean of a medical school was expected to be a leading intellectual who saw the educational mission as primary and who wore the title of dean with pride. Contemporary titles such as chief executive officer and vice chancellor did not exist and would have seemed superfluous if not fatuous. Furthermore, deans were chosen because of leadership qualities defined in the realm of the intellect, not simply the boardroom. I've long bemoaned the fact that today's "deans" no longer read poetry, let alone write poetry; they are expert at creating and staffing epidemics of committees. But Robert Ebert was a dean in the historical sense, if you can liken medical students to monks under the tutelage of their medieval "dean." The episode with Dean Ebert was recorded in an essay titled "Training for Tomorrow's Needs" in the February 25, 1966, issue of *Time* magazine. The manifesto declared, "We are growing intellectually passive . . . much of our time is squandered in academic exercises from which we learn little." My class had taken to recording and transcribing lectures rather than attend, freeing up time to pursue academic interests. This was not a class of rebels. To the contrary, we were seriously committed to our education and our career choice. It is a class that has endowed medicine with major scholars and practitioners, including two Nobel Prize winners (Eric Chivian and Ralph Steinman), many members of national academies, and leading professors in most of the clinical and preclinical disciplines. All we wanted was the freedom to pursue intellectual challenges while we did the donkeywork of assimilating the standard curriculum. For example, we argued that dissecting a cadaver was an antiquated and time-consuming rite of passage; it should be an elective later in the curriculum for those who might be interested in surgery or in doing autopsies. Dean Ebert allowed us the leeway we sought and even went on to create a largely elective preclinical curriculum for the classes to follow.[4] That experiment failed. Nearly all subsequent classes elected gross anatomy and the other subjects traditionally offered in the preclinical years, fearing they would miss something by missing the rite of passage.

There have been many less-dramatic experiments with the standard curriculum, each doomed to succeed in the short term. Any truly meaningful curriculum change would require a change in the culture of the academy; after all, academic medical departments gain more than credence in the academic health center by virtue of their roles, however minor, in educating medical students. Many years ago, over lunch, I asked the late Eugene Stead, the legendary professor of medicine at Duke University Medical Center, why we still have a Department of Biochemistry in our medical schools and a separate Department of Chemistry in arts and sciences when the intellectual purviews overlap to a very large extent, as do their roles in educating Ph.D. candidates. Why not have just a Chemistry Department in arts and sciences and remunerate that department for its input into the education of medical students. Stead's answer was "money." The biochemists vie for grants from the National Institutes of Health, which are more generous, have higher salaries, and cover the full year. Chemists vie for grants from the National Science Foundation, which fall short on all these accounts. The biochemists were not going to abandon the "Sick Citadel"[5] quietly.

Despite many noble initiatives, medical schools are not likely to turn themselves inside out to design a curriculum that takes the foundation for a lifetime of continuing education as its grail. The pressure to do so will have to come from the physicians in practice once they realize that more is expected of them as they progress in their careers—and not just more about less and less. Someday, the "preclinical" curriculum will see graduate clinicians joining students in seminars, each generation helping the other understand what is both interesting and relevant, and why. Or . . . the pragmatists will come to dominate, and "doctors" will be viewed as gatekeepers and technicians rather than humanistic physicians. Heaven forbid; but there are great pressures in this direction today.

Clinical Clerkship

Both the preclinical and clinical curricula suffer from the entropy of balkanization and financing to this day. One reason is that every discipline wants its chance at the students. It's partly an exercise in recruitment of students and partly in self-validation. The result is undercurrents of which few medical students are aware and for which very few are a match.

My first exposure to clinical faculty occurred early in the first year of medical school, when I, like all others in the class, was assigned a mentor. Mine happened to be Vernon Herschel Mark, the chief of neurosurgery at the Harvard Service of Boston City Hospital. I was elated; at that point, I was considering neurosurgery as a career goal.

Dr. Mark put an end to that notion. He was one of the last proponents of "psychosurgery," an invention of neurosurgeons who believed there might be a surgical solution to whatever was deemed an intellectual or psychological disease by those in position to do the deeming. The tragic saga of the "frontal lobotomy" is a legacy of psychosurgery. When it finally became clear that frontal lobotomy created a wretched neurological disease, psychosurgeons became more inventive rather than perspicacious: they tried slicing other parts of the brain. Dr. Mark's particular *cause célèbre* was to try to cure violent behavior with a scalpel. The more he explained and defended his approach, the more I bridled. I brought a deep distrust of moral relativism to our dialogue. We crossed swords; rather, I took my slingshot away and saved its stone for another day and time. I also came away with a fierce belief that ethical issues were as central to medicine as anything science could bring to the bedside.

There was no forum for such matters back then, and no didactic sessions, either. Today, ethical issues are widely acknowledged. Most medical schools offer an ethics course—a week or two in the preclinical years, as if ethics is something discrete to be mastered by students, similar to their taking a brief course in immunology. Of all that is lacking in the education of the physician in medical school and throughout professional life, ethics ranks at the top of my list, along with an understanding of the interactions between life as a patient and life as a person. Ethical challenges are part of the practice of medicine on a daily basis. Professionalism demands they be acknowledged and considered in a transparent way and case by case. I want the entering medical student to be primed for the challenge of confronting the ethical dilemmas of medical practice (if not life). I want the "curriculum in ethics" to be inculcated in the daily discourse at the bedside. No opportunity to question value and values should be missed. I want all this for the sake of the patients of today and of tomorrow. I have a lot of wants.

I began the clinical years with a "clerkship" on the vaunted surgery services at the Massachusetts General Hospital (MGH). It was my first exposure to the MGH; it was everything Parkchester General was not. The institution dripped traditions of clinical excellence. It had earned its reputation as the beacon for postwar Western medicine. It also had a reputation of being haughty, but it never felt so from the inside, even as a medical student. We felt welcomed on the surgical service, a part of the tradition of excellence it boasted. But that clerkship ended whatever vestige of my ambition to be a surgeon had survived Dr. Mark. Surgeons like to do surgery; elite surgeons like to do it better. To a surgeon, dealing with a particular part of a patient who is anesthetized is the best part of a day. Surgical "judgment" includes deciding who needs surgery but rises higher when it comes to deciding how to do the procedure and how to overcome challenges during the operation. I value and appreciate surgical judgment and seek it for my patients who are surgical candidates—but it never fascinated me.

Dr. Mark aside, many elite surgeons were scholars of scope, matches for the likes of a David Seegal. Many were well read and thoughtful. Many were committed to the care of their patients with zeal—during the surgical illness. Few understood that the surgical illness was just one among many events in the patient's life course. Most simply compartmentalized the current admission; all that mattered was to discharge the case as "cured." This all remains true today, as does the notable degree of imperiousness that surgeons seem to emulate. The striking difference today relates to finances. Most of the members of the faculties of elite medical schools throughout the history of American medicine (Western medicine in general) up through the 1960s were men of means, but earnings, investments, wealth, and the like were topics considered too gauche for public discourse. There was pride in volunteerism and philanthropy, as there is today. But today, doctors' lounges, meeting rooms, and, if they remain separated, dining rooms sound like trading floors. Issues relating to income, including that derived from medical practice, are much more likely to dominate conversations than the clinical challenges of the day. I appreciate that fewer people today enter medicine as "men or women of means," and most exit medical school servicing considerable debt, but the din is not conducive to professionalism at any level. Let's bring back the "curbside consults," where trainees can watch mentors teach each other how to be better physicians in public. Today, if two members of the clinical faculty are overheard in the corridor, they are likely to be talking about medical politics and the financial ramifications of health-care reform. The fact that they cannot discuss particular patients in public without violating the ethics of privacy and compliance with HIPAA (the Health Insurance Portability and

Accountability Act of 1996) does not preclude talking about relevant clinical challenges in the abstract.

I was adrift after the surgical rotation at the MGH, going through the motions that year until I landed at the Boston City Hospital (BCH) for my medical rotation. The Harvard Service at the BCH was a two-story building with an enormous open ward on each floor. The BCH was the neighborhood hospital for South Boston, a part of the city populated by working-class Irish immigrant families—"Southies." The open wards were extensions of this community. The patient population was voluminous and very sick. The wards were staffed by a handful of interns, residents, and students supervised by faculty members on the staff of the Thorndike Memorial Laboratory, along with an inadequate number of truly marvelous, committed, and skilled nurses and allied health professionals. There was a division in the tasks for which each profession was primarily responsible, but the division was never inviolate, and if there was a "pecking order," it, too, was anything but inviolate. We all lifted and transferred patients, measured blood pressures, drew bloods, changed linens; whatever was necessary was to be done as expeditiously as possible by whoever was available at the moment. Cohesiveness was the secret to the high level of care afforded these patients. Thorndike faculty members were a special breed. They did not seem to be bothered by the hectic, paint-peeling ambience of a city hospital. Rather, they thrived, joining the residents in orchestrating exemplary care in a teaching setting. Most pursued research careers of international repute. Some became legendary in their disciplines: Charles Davidson in liver disease, James Jandl in hematology, Sidney Ingbar in endocrinology, Derek Denny-Brown in neurology, and Maxwell Finland in infectious diseases, to name a few. The Thorndike glowed with the mystique of its early years; Francis W. Peabody passed the baton of leadership to George Minot, who, along with William Murphy, earned the Nobel Prize for treating pernicious anemia with raw liver. They were followed by William B. Castle, who sorted out why that worked.

To be fair, I should point out that Harvard Medical School was not alone in accumulating laurels by midcentury, just nearly alone. Very few American medical schools had nurtured an academic tradition of this stature. The College of Physicians & Surgeons at Columbia University; the Universities of Pennsylvania, Michigan, Chicago, and

Toronto; Yale; the newcomer Johns Hopkins; and several others come to mind. All these have stories that rival those I am relating about Harvard. Most American medical schools were not advantaged by communities that could afford to support such independent thinking or by faculty members with the personal resources to devote themselves to academic pursuits. Most faced more than enough challenges in recruiting voluntary faculty to help produce practicing physicians. The enormous academic health establishment that has a presence in nearly every state is a triumph of the post-Truman era.

Medical students who applied and were chosen to train at the BCH in its heyday were exceedingly bright and had no need to be coddled as residents. Harvard medical students on rotation at the BCH were welcomed into the flow of the ward to whatever extent they were capable. Some kept up better than others. Thanks to all my years at Parkchester General, the mechanics of patient care (blood drawing, moving patients, doing lab tests, etc.) were second nature. I joined the brotherhood fully, capable of getting the work done efficiently so that I could spend time getting to know the patients and the other physicians and exploring whatever literature might optimize the care of the patient. For students and residents, "time" was not an issue. We had much to do, and we did it. We would help each other, spell each other, and take pride in making another feel competent and look good. Trust me; these were all strong personalities, spirited and ambitious young men (there were very few women medical students and no women residents at the BCH at the time). The driver to cohesiveness was not altruism; the driver was to learn to be a superior physician in the context of a residency in a city hospital knowing full well that few if any would spend their career in such a setting. I remember the residents I worked with fondly. Many have pursued academic careers quite successfully. We have a bond to this day, not just the bond of meeting the challenges of caring for patients in an underfunded, understaffed municipal hospital but of pushing ourselves to do so in a fashion that never lost sight of the human being in each hospital bed. No other "lesson" stands out as comparable in educational value in all four years I spent in medical school. Comforting, crying, and chortling were interventions at least as necessary as any in the pharmacopoeia.

Of course, there is a downside to any culture that demands such an intense and relentless level of performance. Those who can't or won't keep up are dropped from memory, if not from this particular career path. For some, this is tragic; for others, this is the blessing that stimulates their choosing a path for which they are more suited; and for yet others, this is an object lesson in unforgiving cultures. After all, we must also count among these the colleagues, staff, and patients who are not well served. It is not easy to be a patient in an open ward surrounded by hustle, and it is not always therapeutic. It is not easy for some students to learn on the fly. The ambience of the "Harvard Service" on the Thorndike was far from inclusive; the terminal patient and the "weak" student could be left by the wayside.

Residency Training

I left this three-month student clerkship enthralled with the scope of internal medicine and understanding what was expected of me as a student. I was expected to understand the mechanisms of disease, the science of therapy, and the secrets to managing a patient's care in the inpatient setting. I was not expected to "know" my patient. I went about the rest of medical school interested in the potpourri of clerkships and seminars. But I got back on track as an intern and resident on the medical service of the Massachusetts General Hospital. The experience would take the skills and reflexes I started to hone on the Thorndike to new heights.

Titles like "resident" and "house officer" are throwbacks to an earlier time, but only to a generation earlier than mine, when postgraduate training programs required that one be unmarried and reside in-house. Hospitals emerged from Edwardian times with dormitories for nurses and for young doctors in training. Room and board was considered adequate compensation. The dormitories still existed in my day and were used for night call, but none of us lived there, and many of us were married. This slowly dawned on the administration of these teaching hospitals. When I was a rising fourth-year medical student, it was announced that the annual salary for an intern would be raised from $1,000 to $3,000. My wife and I felt flush, so flush that we started our family. So did others in my cohort, and still others got married. It didn't occur to us that the rise in salary did little to abrogate the exhaustion that we would have to surmount while working thirty-six hours out of every forty-eight for most of the next two years.

Internship and residency was demanding, even exhausting, but not brutal in the least for me. It was brutal, however, for my wife, who was de facto a single parent whose husband returned every other evening totally exhausted. I don't know how my wife managed, and managed brilliantly, but I was grateful at the time, and my gratitude has grown over the years. For her, these were a very trying two years, but not for me: I was totally immersed in the care of patients—loving the experience and proud of the reflexes I was developing as a physician. I never felt alone, or lonely, in the hospital. We were a dozen men and one woman in my cohort at the MGH. The emotional, interpersonal ambience of the medical service had much in common with that at Boston City, except there was nothing shabby about the bricks and mortar at the MGH. We cared about each other, helped each other, picked up slack for each other. We knew our patients, the patients of the physicians we were teamed with, and the nursing staff involved in their care. Little was taken for granted, and practically nothing was overlooked. And we were part of a medical community that was immediately available, from other residents to many on the faculty, including those who roamed the corridors at night caring for their own patients.

As was true for most of its peer institutions in that day, the MGH was divided into three hospitals. Each served a different economic stratum. The Bulfinch Building still stands in the center of the institution. Charles Bulfinch was a very prominent Harvard-educated architect of the Federal Period who plied his trade between Boston and Washington. Many a building still stands in testimony to his work, including parts of the U.S. Capitol. The Bullfinch Building at the MGH was the entire MGH when it opened its doors in 1821, the first general hospital in Boston and the third in the country. As is true of its predecessors in Philadelphia and New York, the Bullfinch Building was built to replace the almshouse for the care of Boston's poor; the wealthy were cared for at home. It is a stately, granite, Greek revival structure that was state-of-the art at the time, with flush toilets, central heating, and five usable floors. When I was a resident, the top floor housed the famous "Ether Dome," which had been converted into a charming, intimate auditorium. It was where the first public demonstration of ether as an anesthetic occurred on October 16, 1846. The basement housed "Ward 4," famous as the setting of landmark experiments in metabolism that were undertaken after World War II. The "ground" level was for conference rooms. And the two floor above were each split into open wards, one modified to house the Intensive Care Units of the day. These open wards were structured and staffed similarly to what I described at the Boston City Hospital. However, the Bullfinch was surrounded by other buildings, several of which served different patient populations. The Bullfinch housed "charity" care. The White Building was the surgical building, Phillips House was for the very wealthy, and the Baker Pavilion was for those with health insurance. Patients in the latter two facilities had private doctors and a more-distant relationship to the residents and the teaching agenda. Bullfinch was the center of that activity. In an earlier book,[6] I used the transition in the structure of the MGH in the 1960s to illustrate the transition to an insured patient population that followed the passing of Medicare. "Charity care" largely disappeared, and over time, the Bullfinch Building came to be yet another home for wayward administrators.

As mentioned, there were about a dozen in my cohort. That means there were three dozen medical residents staffing the medical service (including the emergency ward and Intensive Care Units) at any given time for a very large hospital with a very busy emergency service serving an inner city.[7] Today, the corps of medicine residents numbers 178. The increase is not proportional to the increase in bed capacity, though it does correlate with the turnover. The same is true for all major teaching hospitals, including UNC Hospitals. In the 1960s, residents and students drew bloods, rounded repeatedly, met with nurses who were actually caring for patients directly and dispensing medicines, checked and rechecked and routinely rewrote hospital orders, and managed to cover busy wards every other night. There was a great deal of camaraderie. Some felt humbled by the responsibilities, some felt insecure, and some felt overwhelmed. None suffered feelings of inadequacy alone; there was an intimacy to these years in the "trenches." The cohort could and did compensate for members who had physical impairments and for those who felt like fish out of water. Some redirected their career paths away from the clinical arena, often to highly productive research careers. My cohort produced many a world-class scholar in basic sciences, including a Nobel Prize winner, the dean of arts and sciences at an Ivy League university, and senior laboratory scientists at the National Institutes of Health and elsewhere, as well as many a professor in a clinical discipline. This was not a "one size fits all" environment. It was a time when each of us learned the care of the patient with every fiber in our bodies and appreciated those who aspired to excellence in that arena. And each of us welcomed and valued any assistance our colleagues and mentors offered—and offer they did.

The intellectual ambience of the medical service was spectacular. Our charts and conferences were challenging discussions of the limitations of certainty regarding diseases and treatment. The weekly "Allen Street" conference was a no-holds-barred discussion of what went wrong with/for patients that week (the conference was named for the street used by hearses to access the hospital morgue). None of us had the energy to even consider supplementing our meager salaries by "moonlighting" when we were off duty. Then again, we were not burdened with the inordinate debt many American physicians accumulate today in paying college and medical school tuitions. We made do and had fun doing so. The learning curve was very steep, and the "clinical reflexes" that resulted are indelible.

All of this is looked upon by the residents and the professional educators of today as a dark age, a time when exhausted young physicians were overburdened with responsibility and therefore potentially dangerous. The reaction includes a mandate to limit hours spent in the hospital, the result of which is lonely residents, fragmented care, and no demonstrable improvement in patient outcomes, even in the summer months when the new interns come aboard. Furthermore, there is not only a premium on getting the resident home on time; there is also tremendous pressure to discharge the patient as soon as possible. Camaraderie is the least of the losses for the residency experience; intellectual content is a shadow of what it was. That is all too obvious in the quality of the charting, the conduct of rounds, and the content of conferences. This is but one of many "prices" corporatization levied on health care and that will occupy us in detail in later chapters.

We should have known better. The Council of Europe in Brussels issued a directive in 1998 restricting time at work to forty-eight hours per week for all employees, including medical professionals. There have been many studies of the effect of this restriction on the quality of resident education in the United Kingdom; only one suggested any degree of improvement.[8] The demonstration of an improvement in patient outcomes is similarly elusive. What is not elusive is the increasing reliance on physicians who accept short-term employment and the general consensus that patient care has suffered by these changes in the culture of inpatient caring.[9]

There is nothing "wrong" with immersing oneself during formative years to gain skills that will underpin professional excellence going forward. We applaud this in professional musicians, professional athletes, clergy, and chefs. Why not "doctors"? Because, some argue, they are overworked and therefore less keen in performing their task. But that is said by individuals who do not understand the training paradigm of the American teaching hospitals of the 1960s, a paradigm that fostered as much concern among the trainees for each other as for their charges. That is lost today, but hopefully not irretrievably lost. The academic medical centers of 1960 America were both academic and medical and remain a gold standard for medical education to this day.

Massachusetts General Hospital in the 1960s

Prior to World War II, American medicine suffered from an inferiority complex. In the eighteenth and nineteenth centuries, French medicine was considered preeminent. Some features of American medicine today are borrowed from French traditions. For example, "Grand Rounds" can trace its roots to the amphitheater in the medical school in Montpelier, where Rabelais held forth in the sixteenth century. But by the turn of the twentieth century, Prussian medicine had risen to preeminence. French humanist traditions that valued keen observation of the human condition and the holistic notion of *terrain* seemed antiquated in light of the burgeoning reductionistic but relevant biological science that poured forth from the laboratories of Robert Koch, Paul Ehrlich, Otto Wallach, Fritz Haber, Otto Meyerhof, Karl Landsteiner, Otto Warburg, and many others. Nearly all American notables had felt that postgraduate studies in Berlin were necessary if they were to realize their ambitions. They returned home armed with the scientific method and imbued with scientific zeal. But American medicine was too entrenched in its humanistic traditions to abandon the bedside. The American old guard championed a balance between science and humanism. Those who returned having received training in the Prussian approach assumed this mantle. The writings by James Putnam, William Osler, and Francis Peabody quoted earlier bear witness to this. American academics started to apply the new scientific methodology at the bedside and ushered in a most extraordinary chapter in medical history; the pathophysiology of disease was moved from the haze of theory to the domain of evidence.

The Massachusetts General Hospital was basking in international renown prior to the turn of the century. After all, in addition to its "Ether Dome" demonstration of 1846, in 1886 Reginald Fitz had managed to sort "appendicitis" from the clinical confusion about causes of abdominal pain. These and several other diagnostic and even therapeutic (mainly surgical) breakthroughs positioned the MGH among the handful of American institutions of international repute. However, it was the application of scientific methods to the study of illness that would catapult the MGH and its few sister American research hospitals to the forefront of medical science and medical care by midcentury. This was the birthing of the "clinical investigator" and the creation of the modern academic hospital. By midcentury, American medicine had vaulted to such preeminence that physicians from abroad aspired to a "BTA" (Been to America) as a prerequisite to advancement in their own countries. BTA remains a credential to this day.

The prototypical setting for clinical investigation at the start of this era was "Ward 4," an inpatient corridor in the basement of the Bullfinch Building at the MGH. Patients were admitted to Ward 4 by their physicians for the purpose of studying the causes of their diseases. In Ward 4, these clinical investigators could control diet if appropriate and measure all sorts of chemicals in body fluids in a controlled fashion. Thanks to the genius of the likes of Joseph Aub and Fuller Albright, modern endocrinology was born in this hallowed basement. Ward 4 was the model for "'Clinical Research Units" in many teaching hospitals to follow and for the Clinical Center at the National Institutes of Health. Within a generation or two, the vein of normal physiology and pathophysiology that required a living subject had been thoroughly mined. The next frontiers were back in the laboratory. These special research beds still exist but are now largely dedicated to derivative science, studies analyzing the relevance of laboratory-derived insights, including drug trials and other "translational research." But in the 1960s, translational research that included systematic testing of therapeutic interventions was still in its infancy.

There was another contribution of this era of innovative clinical investigation that has at least as much of a far-reaching impact. The dialogue at the bedside of the ill patient was changed. No longer was "we see that" or "that's what we always do" considered a demonstration of authority; it was considered merely a default when there was nothing better to consider. Bedside teaching was rich with discussions of the limitations of understanding of the presenting complaints, the diagnosis, the mechanism of disease, and the rationale for treatment. Reading and discussing the relevant literature became de rigueur. Conferences around a table or around the bedside were Socratic. And notes in charts were written to record progress and thinking, often with references, so that another physician or student could readily and fully understand the patient's status. The "teaching hospital" became the center of a great deal of intellectual excitement that played out at the bedside. The goal was optimal care for the patient in that bed. If there was any urgency, it was dictated by the pace of the patient's illness and not the pace of processing the admission.

While clinical scholarship, bedside teaching, and inpatient care flourished in the 1960s, the care of the patient after discharge and, for that matter, the care of the person yet to be ill was as uneven as ever. This was reflected in the organization of elite institutions such as the MGH. As I touched on earlier, the MGH was actually three hospitals: the Phillips House, the Baker Pavilion, and the Bullfinch. The Phillips House contained elegantly appointed private rooms dedicated to the care of the rich and powerful. Only their private physicians were allowed to orchestrate their care. In fact, the physician's name, not the patient's, was emblazoned on the medical records. House officers (and students) were welcome in the Phillips House only by invitation, which usually was precipitated by an emergency. The Phillips House was as private a hospital as one can imagine. Unlike Parkchester General and its ilk, the Phillips House was a hospital where the private physicians could call upon consultants and facilities of the larger institution and thereby afford their coddled patients the best care available. Of course, that required private physicians whose skills lived up to that promise. Peer review and peer pressure were not built into the Phillips House as they were elsewhere at the MGH.

Most Americans, employed or not, young or old, had no health insurance in that era. They might be able to afford an office visit or even a house call, since these fees were within reach for the average family. Few had the resources to pay for hospitalization and inpatient procedures. The larger institutions developed "ward services," which were underwritten by government, as for Boston City Hospital, or by philanthropists and other sources for a not-for-profit private hospital like the MGH. In the 1960s, the Bullfinch Building was MGH's medical ward service, with several floors of open wards not very different from the Boston City Hospital. The ward service was the kingdom of the residents and of the medical students that followed in their wake. Staff physicians who were pursuing academic careers, as with the staff of the Thorndike at the BCH, took month-long stints as "attending physician" to supervise the resident staff on a particular ward. Teaching rounds were frequent, some with and some without faculty presence. Regardless, attending physicians were at the beck and call of the residents. The Bullfinch roiled with enthusiasm, scholarly conversation and a concerted effort to do the best for each patient. At discharge, patients were offered appointments in clinics held by residents; some accepted, while others returned to their neighborhood resources.

The Baker Pavilion had semiprivate rooms occupied by the few patients who could afford them and the growing number who could afford health insurance or, more likely, were provided health insurance by their employer. All had a private physician who was in charge of their care and received remuneration for his efforts. Residents and students were part of the staffing of the Baker Pavilion, working for/with the private physicians. Faculty appeared each day to round with the residents and students as an academic exercise to supplement whatever information was forthcoming from the private physicians and to make certain that the patient care they participated in was consonant with the educational goals of the "teaching hospital." Admitting privileges to the Baker Pavilion (and Phillips House) were sought after by private practitioners. Those granted such privileges had impressive credentials, often including having trained at an elite teaching hospital.

By the end of the 1960s, the American "teaching hospital" was a high point in the history of medical education. It took the understanding and treatment of disease from pronouncement and opinion to substantive discussion. It elevated the "doctor" from empiricist to scholar.

It set goals for bedside teaching that reverberated around the United States and abroad. But it also had its downsides. The teaching hospital tended to objectify patients, turning them into examples of disease rather than emphasizing their nobility and humanity. It generally ignored the psychosocial context in which they suffered. And it was overtly stratified by socioeconomic status.

Even though the American teaching hospital of the 1960s was the creation of a nation that eschewed the European precedents for a national health-insurance scheme, it was not driven by profit. It was succored by the quest for clinical excellence. And it trained the next generation of "doctors" in that ethos.

CHAPTER THREE

The Golden Age That *Wasn't*

The 1970s and 1980s

Many aspects of medicine were refashioned during the 1970s, the decade of transition. America had commenced its first-ever important assault on its have-and-have-not stratification of health care by enacting Medicare legislation in 1965. The extramural programs of the National Institutes of Health fostered the development of a full-time academic establishment in medical schools across the nation. Community-based medical schools grew academic teaching hospitals and research establishments. The age seemed particularly "golden" from the perspective of "the doctor," who abandoned a highly respected, traditional cottage industry to commence ascending toward the pinnacle of national influence as the driving force behind the modern American academic hospital. Furthermore, such hospitals were no longer the pride of a few elite institutions but the template for medical education across the country and the envy of the industrialized world. In the chapters that follow, we will learn how the academic teaching hospital transformed into the modern academic health center in which both the education of the physician and the care of the patient are no longer top priorities.

Double-Edged Swords

The dramatic developments in diagnosis and therapy that occurred in the 1970s reverberate to this day. The legacy of the American teaching hospital, which we will soon examine, is mixed. The salutary legacy is obvious and celebrated to this day; it's the downsides that are little appreciated. There remains much to be done about disparities in access to health care and unevenness in the quality of care even today, despite the Affordable Care Act. However, the emphasis on disparities in access has obscured the even-more-pressing malevolence of disparities in health in the first place. It turns out that one's station in life, the degree to which one feels disaffected or disallowed, is a far greater determinant of health than access to health care or provision of health care. The emphasis on access to health care is missing the forest for the trees, which is not to say that none of the trees are worthy of attention.

Furthermore, the burgeoning of the research-based academy has become an end in itself. The academic health centers that proliferated are progressively less and less academic and less and less committed to health or health care. They are cumbersome, self-serving enterprises, though some of their accomplishments certainly are important for those who are ill and those who are well.

I have discussed both of these points in great detail in previous works.[1] Here, we will examine the collateral damage that was done to the "doctor" and the doctor-patient relationship by this dialectic. The 1970s saw the construction of a new, peculiarly American form of health-care system. The notion that American medicine was an altruistic profession was superseded by a proud new institutionalized medicine supported by several costly and discrete pillars looking down and over the people it was meant to serve. In this institution, the "doctor" is but one of the potentates with great wealth and independence. The other potentates were recruited from the infrastructure and promoted to positions of influence. The supporting pillars were built on tenuous footings that proved vulnerable to the shifting sands of the late twentieth century. Now they are at risk of crumbling altogether—and the risk is imminent.

Medicare

Elsewhere, I have detailed the bumpy, if not tortuous, political road that President Lyndon Johnson traveled before he could sign Title XVIII of the Social Security Act into law in 1965, thereby creating Medicare. Of all the wheeling-and-dealing required, one compromise in particular has had a lasting effect on the role of the American doctor in society. Organized medicine, mainly by virtue of the power of the American Medical Association (AMA) at that time, decried

Medicare as a landfall for "socialized medicine." This was the era of the "cold war," and the notion of anything socialized enflamed the body politic. The term "socialized" was coined advisedly; calling it a "national health insurance scheme," as was common in Europe, would not have served the AMA's political agenda nearly as well. The fear of socialization was central in all the debates. American doctors were not willing to be government employees, in fact or de facto, and demanded a codicil to that effect as a concession. The AMA and the Johnson administration came to a compromise that allowed for the enactment of Title XVIII; the legislation would stipulate the autonomy of physicians in caring for the elderly. The AMA was granted the responsibility for determining what services doctors would provide and the "customary and usual" charge for any such service. This compromise placed a major moral imperative on the collective shoulders of the medical profession. Doctors were entrusted to consider the welfare of the patient as the sole reason for indemnifying any service and to consider their fee structure in the context of the common good. Medicine is to be first and foremost a "service profession." The AMA's Code of Medical Ethics in 1957 stipulated that medical fees must be on a sliding scale "commensurate with the services rendered and the patient's ability to pay." By 1980, the code supplanted the sliding scale with the language of Medicare: customary, usual, and reasonable.

Medicare provided the missing piece of a magna carta for American doctors, who had collectively bridled at any incursion on their autonomy. They already controlled licensure in each state and, more important, could define who did not deserve medical licensure. They could also define what they were licensed to do and what others could not (see chapter 1). Now under Medicare, they could define the dollar amount they would be reimbursed if they provided care for the elderly under contract to the federal government. My profession—the profession whose potential I feel bound to champion—had abandoned such indefensible idioms as "soaking the rich" and "charity care." Instead, it had positioned itself beneath Damocles's sword. The meager financial resources of the elderly had been replaced by the federal coffer. The profession would need a polished moral compass in defining a usual, customary, and reasonable fee structure, or the "doctor" could become a card-carrying member of an exclusive, exploitive, self-serving guild.

If the profession did not monitor its own enthusiasm, misguided treatments could compete with appropriate care for reimbursement.

The process by which fees-for-services are determined by physicians under Medicare was adopted, largely unchanged and often by dint of state legislation, for fee schedules under employer-sponsored health-insurance plans and for private policies held by individuals. Such policies were becoming commonplace by the 1970s and rapidly provided a pocket nearly as deep as the federal coffer. Private health insurance was a benefit almost exclusively afforded those who worked for a larger employer. Taking workers' compensation indemnity schemes as the precedent, these larger employers found it seductive to "self-insure." That means they paid all medical expenses out of pocket and turned to private health-insurance companies to administer the beneficence under a "cost plus" agreement. Hence, the more money flowing through the system, the more that is retained by the administering insurance company. For the insurance company, there is an obvious disincentive to promulgate efficiency at any level. As long as the employer could afford to pay, greater charges result in merriment for all the purveyors and other "stakeholders." Medicare produced the perfect conditions for a growth in the "health-care dollar" in the United States. The clouds collected in the 1970s, and the storm unleashed through the 1980s, bloating the "health-care dollar" at a rate that has outstripped all other resource-advantaged countries.

Without such underwriting, the theories underlying interventional cardiology and cardiovascular surgery might have remained untested in the 1970s; instead, these fields exploded, particularly in the United States. I recall the debate in 1973 at the Massachusetts General Hospital regarding coronary artery bypass grafting for coronary artery disease. It was a heady time: in twenty years, anesthesiology had advanced from dripping ether onto face masks to sophisticated intubation and life-support procedures that made prolonged and aggressive surgery possible. In twenty years, cardiac surgery had advanced from blindly cutting a fused heart valve with a blade attached to the surgeon's finger to replacing the valve while the patient's circulation was supported by a pump on the floor.

But there are only so many valves that needed replacement; there are many, many more patients with atherosclerotic plaques plugging their coronary arteries that seemed ripe for bypassing. The cardiovascular surgeons at the Massachusetts General Hospital were a match for the technical demands of the bypassing but raised concerns as to whether it would help. Those concerns were no match for the zeal of others, notably the surgeons at the Cleveland Clinic, who were growing an enterprise with great visibility and profitability. Every major hospital, and many not so major, was soon developing the teams and hardware to join in the scramble.[2] By the end of the 1970s, American surgeons were performing over 100,000 coronary artery bypass grafting procedures a year, and by the end of the 1980s, they were performing over half a million. All this is supported by Medicare for the elderly, Medicaid for the poor, private health insurance for most others, and mounting debt for the uninsured. It continues apace, accompanied by over a million alternative procedures (various forms of angioplasty and stenting) each year. It continues apace despite the prescient concerns of the cardiac surgeons in 1973; demonstrable benefit of these procedures is elusive in scientific testing, except for a tiny subset.[3]

Do not misunderstand me. Medicare was a double-edged sword, a watershed in American communitarian ethics. No longer would the elderly in America fear dying destitute and forlorn from diseases that could be effectively treated or from illnesses that could be effectively managed. If there is anything wrong with providing such assurance, it is that America lagged behind the rest of the industrialized world by half a century in providing for its ill elderly. The devil of Medicare is in its details regarding determination of appropriateness of care and remuneration for care. But its beneficence was obvious soon after enactment. The escalation in the transfer of wealth it underwrote that did not benefit the insured was less obvious at the outset. It did not take hold for a decade and now is simply uncontrollable and unconscionable.

The Effect of Medicare on Clinical Training

The ward services described previously were rapidly replaced across the country by semiprivate rooms, as is stipulated for full Medicare reimbursement. Many elderly patients who would have been "charity cases" became a source of income for public and private hospitals. Similarly, physicians donating their time to charity care became an antiquated notion when it came to elderly patients. In the academic hospitals, attending physicians were generating income in the course of supervising the care of elderly Medicare recipients, unless another private practitioner was the attending of record. Even trainees were generating income: Medicare reimbursement schemes allowed greater charges for a stay in a teaching hospital to subsidize the supplementary care afforded by physicians in training. The cozy arrangement that reimbursed teaching hospitals for the care delivered by teachers and by trainees simultaneously was to have a comeuppance, but in the 1970s, it totally changed the financial model of the teaching hospital. Now there was money to spare.

American hospitals in the early 1970s were just that—hospitals. The leadership was dominated by the medical staff. Boards of leading citizens provided community input, sometimes expert management and business skills, and often did so gratis. Administration was lean, and administrative roles were clearly defined. "Dietary" prepared meals, "purchasing" purchased, "nursing" nursed, and the "pharmacy" dispensed. Everyone knew their role in making the hospital function as a facility that supported the needs of inpatient care. Yes, there were errors and inefficiencies, but no one viewed the hospital as a factory producing widgets with "six sigma" reliability. The hospital was an extension of the community of caring, not a citadel. Medicare reimbursement was viewed as a means for hospitals to serve a larger segment of the population. The culture was little changed, including the role of the "doctor," well into the 1970s, except that fee-for-service largely supplanted charity care on open wards.

Clinical Center of the National Institutes of Health

The 1970s saw the escalation of the war in Vietnam leading up to the fall of Saigon in 1975. All young men had to confront the likelihood of being drafted, but not all young physicians did; for them, service was mandatory. However, it could be postponed until medical school and postgraduate training were completed. There were alternatives to military service, including obtaining a commission in the Public Health Service and, more particularly, a commission as a public health officer assigned to the National Institutes of Health (NIH) or the Centers for Disease Control (CDC). These were desirable and highly competitive alternatives to service in the active military. The result was that some of the most accomplished graduates of the most prestigious medical schools and residencies found themselves spending two years or more working in laboratories at the NIH or in the programs of the CDC. Most who gained entry to the NIH served as clinical associates, who were chosen to work in particular laboratories and to care for patients who volunteered to participate in related clinical research protocols. Many of these volunteer patients were admitted to the Clinical Center of the NIH with serious illnesses. The Warren Grant Magnuson Clinical Center opened in 1953 and was greatly expanded in 2005 with the addition of the Mark O. Hatfield Clinical Research Center. The Clinical Center was, and is, the largest research hospital in the world. It is on the campus of the NIH in Bethesda, Maryland, and designed to undertake clinical research to complement the laboratory research in the adjacent buildings. It is an enormous "Ward 4."

Upon completion of their two-year obligation, some of the commissioned public health officers stayed on at the NIH or CDC, and some pursued research or administrative careers elsewhere. Most entered the inactive reserve and returned to civilian settings to complete their specialty and subspecialty training. This is the pool of talent that was to spread across the country to staff the expanding medical schools and medical faculties of the 1970s and 1980s. They were the prototypical "three-legged stools" of American academic medicine: researchers, clinicians, and academic administrators all wrapped into one. They determined the course of American academic medicine for forty years and are its senior citizenry today. I am one of them, except I never grew, or wanted to grow, an administrative leg. Furthermore, very few had three sturdy legs, and some had three rickety ones. Without question, this cohort was the vanguard of the mind-boggling advances in scientific medicine that moved the care of the patient and the education of the clinician into the modern age. It may be the sole beneficence of the war in Vietnam, albeit unintended and unexpected. But it had downsides, too. This is a cohort that came to exalt administrative power and applaud grantsmanship, while denigrating excellence in bedside teaching as less important than research and touting excellence in clinical care as necessary to maintain cash flow and not the pinnacle of medical professionalism.[4] This is one stain on American medicine that would facilitate the development of corporate medicine by the turn of the century.[5]

Private Practice

Since completing my training in the early 1970s, I have been employed by the state of North Carolina as a member of the faculty of the School of Medicine at the University of North Carolina and a member of the attending staff of its associated hospital. I am salaried; my patients are charged the "customary" fees and receipts disappear into the maw of this complex organization. I know a great deal about the UNC maw and more than a little about similar academic health centers. This perspective colors my writing. It also advantages my writing, as the "health center" in general, and the "academic health center" in particular, has superseded private practice as the embodiment of American medicine.

What I know about private practice in the 1950s reflects what I saw in Parkchester General Hospital and in my father's office. I learned what I know about private practice in the 1970s and 1980s from former students and other colleagues who chose to pursue their careers in such settings. Several started out on their own, or with a couple of colleagues. Others joined established groups. All had the rude awakening in confronting the "business" of running a private practice. Most managed. Billing, record keeping, and staffing were easy to get the hang of because they were straightforward. Making ends meet in an office-based practice required some hustling, much networking, and personal drive. Making ends meet in a practice that had ancillary income from specialized procedures was not an issue; cardiologists, nephrologists, ophthalmologists, surgeons, and others had sources of income that made the office practice a secondary source, though necessary to generate the traffic. There were choices, such as whether to support the profitable though increasingly tightly regulated in-office laboratory or x-ray suite. But physicians in private practice largely knew the pleasures of a comfortable income or more and the gratifications derived from autonomy, peer interactions, wide respect, and the opportunity to offer as much quality of care as they were capable. The pleasures of private practice began to erode in the 1990s and today are few and far between for reasons that will occupy us later.

Continuing Medical Education (CME) was not compulsory or institutionalized; it was something that physicians sought out. The AMA didn't coin the term CME until 1959 and made its first foray into the business of accrediting CME providers several years later. I remember going to the dean's office in 1975 with the idea of offering an annual update in rheumatology. The idea was applauded and supported. I was told that we needed to schedule near the weekend and to charge tuition in order to appeal to the target we sought—the practicing physician. The former related to their tight schedules, the latter because doctors then thought that postgraduate education is more valuable if they have to pay out of pocket. I ran this course for three years successfully in terms of size of the audience and camaraderie; we seldom have any data as to whether CME actually changes the thinking or practice of participants. There have been systematic studies about that, with results that are daunting. We stopped the course after three years, in part because of the effort it took on my part but in greater part because of the growing competition. By 1980 the corps of "detail" personnel, a euphemism for sales force, supported by the pharmaceutical industry had grown so large that all in private practice could expect a frequent visit from a smiling young person who was willing to leave samples of drugs and explain over lunch or dinner why these samples were the latest and best. Furthermore, the pharmaceutical industry was developing speakers' bureaus and sponsoring CME exercises that were convenient and often held in enticing locales. The programs always included talks by academics without conflicts of interest and talks by academics with conflicts of interest. Early on, few were concerned whether the audience could readily distinguish between education and marketing in this format. In the 1970s, I agreed to speak at several such CME exercises for Merck, and then I resigned from their "Speakers Bureau," never to participate again as a speaker or an attendee. I made my reservations known in national meetings in the 1980s and in publications, including my early books on occupational musculoskeletal disorders.

CME would become an industry unto itself by the start of this century, and we will have more to say about it in later chapters. But my condemnation of conflicts of interest in the course of patient care has grown ever more strident, even in editorials invited by editors of AMA publications.[6] If a physician is aware of a conflict of interest relevant to a given patient's care, admitting to it and simply carrying on is fatuous. The only defensible action is to refer the patient to a physician whose judgment is not as likely to be tainted.

North Carolina Memorial Hospital

The past century has seen waves of new medical schools, and unlike the days of Flexner when many were forced to close, most are here to stay. One wave followed on the heels of World War II when veterans were returning and settling across the country. The same mindset that caused Harry Truman to create the modern NIH, Clinical Center and all, applied to the sparse and spare state of medical education away from the elite centers. State and federal moneys were expended to create new medical schools and academic hospitals across the country in the Flexnerian mold: the University of Washington, the University of Colorado, the University of Texas Southwestern, the University of California–San Diego, and many others were either founded or greatly expanded and modified. These joined the small cadre of old-line prestigious medical schools as the flagships of the new American institution of medicine. All of them were charged, endowed, and funded to serve the "three-legged chair" mantra. Not surprisingly, all of them were to recruit heavily from the NIH's alumni pool of clinical associates.

The University of North Carolina School of Medicine was founded in the nineteenth century and remained a two-year medical school until 1954. That means it offered a preclinical education; its graduates would go elsewhere for their clinical years. Many from southern preclinical medical schools headed north to Philadelphia and the Jefferson Medical College. There, they completed the clinical years and earned an M.D. degree. That changed in 1954, when the medical school in Chapel Hill started to offer the M.D. In order for this transition to be possible, a number of farsighted legislators and one very farsighted dean had to negotiate turbulent political waters. They were successful, and the state opened the 400-bed North Carolina Memorial Hospital in 1952. Dean Walter Reece Berryhill oversaw the transition of the medical school and the opening of an academic hospital. The background he brought to this leadership role was that he had run the student health service at the university—not much preparation then or now. But he had exquisite leadership skills, best exemplified by the fact that he recruited men who were far more accomplished than he to lead the various departments of the new academic health center. Then he nurtured and supported their efforts, all the while staying out of the spotlight and largely out of their way. Few deans today are leaders in this sense.

I joined the faculty of the University of North Carolina's School of Medicine in 1973. By then, the early growth pains had passed, and the institution was strutting, proudly taking its place in the front ranks of its cohort. All sorts of "three-legged stools" were recruited, and most were placed in a position to garner external funding for their research and clinical income from their bedside activities. The hospital is situated in Chapel Hill, a university town with very few of the medical challenges that characterize the urban settings of most academic health centers. Private practices were few and far between, and the Emergency Department was relatively calm and quiet. Most patients were North Carolinians referred from a distance either because they were quite ill or quite poor, and often both. Medicine in the state was dominated by the private practitioners, many with UNC ties. Fee-for-service was the standard for remuneration. The "carriage trade" was treated in community hospitals or, if the patient or the doctor thought it necessary, sent to a particular consultant at UNC (or neighboring Duke University Medical Center). The 200-year-old university and its School of Medicine painted Chapel Hill with a patina of noblesse oblige more pervasively than I saw anywhere in New Haven or Boston.

North Carolina was, and is, a reprehensibly stratified state that ranks low among U.S. states in per capita income and most of the attributes that are considered progressive. But it is a beautiful state with an advantaged minority that takes such pride in founding the nation's first state university that it supports UNC handsomely, subsidizing tuitions, expanding and maintaining a gorgeous campus, and underwriting its academic health center. This tradition is not surviving recent political contingencies unscathed, but it is still far from extinguished. UNC was wealthy enough to invite me to take my career in any direction I saw fit without constraining my investigative interests to projects that lent themselves to extramural funding. I have never regretted the decision to leave Boston for Chapel Hill, and I have enjoyed over forty years of a thriving family and productive career free from many of the hassles of urban living, commuting in particular. Professionally, the greatest gift UNC has given me is a setting in which I could command the time to reflect on the meanings of medicine, illness, and much more. A career of the breadth I have pursued would not otherwise have been possible. This is not to say that my relationship with the administration of the UNC School of Medicine has been nurturing in either direction; rather, we've spent most of the forty years at loggerheads. But even that has been informative, part of the mix of exposures and experiences that nurtured this book and my earlier books. However, in all my writing and lecturing, I do my best to avoid pointing fingers at individuals or individual institutions. The UNC School of Medicine has had a relatively unfettered ride through the history of American academic medicine over the past forty years without distinguishing itself as an innovator or a Luddite—just mainstream, for better and for worse.

For the first decade or so of my career at UNC, I elected to participate in preclinical teaching. I was part of the team that taught immunology to the first-year class and the "Musculoskeletal System" to the second-year class. I mentioned my thoughts about preclinical teaching in passing above. However, my principal role as a medical educator has been in the clinical arena.

Clinical Education

I am a committed clinical educator. I had role models at Boston City and MGH when I was a medical student and resident. One of the most influential was Professor Daniel Federman, then at the MGH, who seemed to have an unending fund of knowledge and a natural ability to hold forth extemporaneously at the bedside in discourse that was relevant to the particular patient and in language that was accessible to all levels of student—and to the patient. His greatest gift to me was the knowledge that there is no such thing as a born educator. One might be born with the proclivity, but the skills must be acquired. He said that there was nothing extemporaneous about his teaching. He read assiduously and structured his recall to serve his role as a teacher.

My first stint as a clinical teacher (the "attending") on a medical service occurred in the early 1970s, when I was a clinical associate at the NIH. I volunteered to attend at Georgetown Medical School several months a year. I thrived doing so but came away with two unsettling, though valuable, insights. I consider the "attending" function to be the pinnacle of clinical education, yet Georgetown's priorities were such that they would spare their faculty the burden and choose me, although only two intensive years of exposure separated me from my most senior students. The other insight was that my research supervisors at the NIH considered this a lesser endeavor than time in the laboratory and begrudgingly tolerated my absences. Clearly, early in the 1970s, clinical teaching was becoming a stepchild in the American institution of medicine. A decade later, I was decrying this development in publications, but it took that decade for me to understand its depth and scope.

Clinical teaching was valued at North Carolina Memorial Hospital in the 1970s and 1980s. It was required of essentially all the clinical faculty in all the clinical departments, from anesthesia to urology. Perhaps its greatest value to the hospital was related to the income it generated. There was trivial participation by private practitioners at North Carolina Memorial Hospital; essentially, all clinicians were full-time employees on fixed salary. The money to pay us came from several pots: the state contribution to medical education, the salary we were paid by the NIH as part of our research grants, and the money we generated as physicians of record when we were teaching. Rapidly, the leadership realized that state money could be discretionary if it was not necessary to support faculty. Furthermore, it was realized that clinical income also could become discretionary if it flowed into hospital coffers at a rate that exceeded salary requirements. The trick was to create the coffers for clinical income; UNC's was then called "Physicians & Associates" (P&A), which was the entity that employed the clinical faculty as a form of group practice. P&A bills Medicare, Medicaid, private insurers, and patients for our clinical services. P&A is then tithed for all sorts of "administrative" purposes, from the actual administration of P&A to administrators less directly involved (such as the exploding minions of hospital administrators, deans, and the like). "Clinical income" was the engine that grew clinical departments in most medical schools; new faculty could be the source of their own salaries and more.

As an aside, extramural grants from the NIH and elsewhere also contributed to growing the administration in that these grants provided "indirect costs" for this purpose. "Indirect costs" are a sum that is negotiated institution by institution, generally some 50 percent of the "direct costs" though sometimes as much as 100 percent. So if an investigator was awarded a $1 million grant to support the salaries of the personnel involved in the research and the expenses incurred in carrying on the research, the investigator's institution would receive an additional sum, a half million or more, to provide and maintain the necessary infrastructure—everything from lighting and cleaning the buildings to administrative support.

Taking advantage of clinical income became common to all medical schools once "charity care" was indemnified by Medicare and Medicaid. For an institution like UNC, there were no private doctors spoiling that party. Rapidly, the infrastructure became the superstructure of the institution, and clinical teachers were valued primarily for clinical income. Whether they were good teachers or even exemplary clinicians was really not relevant to the administration; you were as good as your clinical income, and it didn't matter who you were.

But clinical excellence was not overlooked by the clinical faculty, and teaching was valued by those who wanted to learn. There was enough money floating around that the size of one's grant or the amount of clinical income that one generated increased one's salary but not necessarily one's prestige. The future of clinical teaching and clinical excellence in this milieu was readily predictable by 1980 and came to pass in the 1990s, as we will discuss in the next chapter.

Teaching at the Bedside

The dichotomy between inpatient and outpatient teaching dates back to the development of the modern medical school a century ago. Clinical education was moved entirely inside the institution and largely onto the ward service. Office-based practice developed either in the private sector or in public-sector "clinics" that were often attached to public hospitals, such as the one at Morrisania Hospital described in chapter 1. Regardless, outpatient care was largely distant from the educational establishment. There was a token effort to provide postgraduate trainees, residents and specialty fellows, with some outpatient clinical exposure. When patients were discharged from the ward services, they were often offered the option of follow-up appointments in the resident's clinic. In my day, residents tore themselves away from the bustle and demands of taking care of inpatients to see follow-up patients in "their" clinic a morning each week. They did the best they could, either relying on their own devices or, if necessary, asking other residents or even faculty for assistance in patient care. The "clinic" was an appendage to the central educational and patient-care role of the inpatient services of teaching hospitals. The exception related to specialty care.

A day on a teaching inpatient service in the 1970s and 1980s varied from institution to institution and from service to service. The surgeons started early, rounded quite early, and then abandoned the bedside for the operating room for a large part of most days, leaving whoever was available and/or low on the totem pole to mind the shop until they emerged after their cases were done. As every medical student will attest, few were lower on the surgical totem pole than the third- or fourth-year year student on rotation through the service. Teaching on the surgical service, then and now, is very much directed to the real-time needs of the particular patients—their wounds and surgical complications. The indication for the surgery was accepted after the fact. The high point of the day was in the operating room during the operation; what happened before and after was considered as issues in process, not prowess. Follow-up appointments in surgical clinics were similarly directed and considered to be part of the process on the route toward a patient being discharged as "cured."

The aura of the modern surgical service, its public image, was established in this time period. It is the turf of the highly efficient, heroic surgeon who, surrounded by acolytes, practices by the "cut is to cure" mantra and is worthy of adulation and generous compensation. Students and residents lined up by height and marched to the drum of seniority. In institutions where private-practice surgeons had admitting privileges, they ascended to the top of the totem for their own patient. If nothing else, a well-functioning surgical service had the esprit of a military unit. The appeal of such ambience was as much a draw toward surgery as a career as the technical and emotional challenges of deciding to operate and then operating successfully.

The elite surgical training programs were as tightly run in terms of quality of care as they were in terms of quantity of procedures. It was customary to have a weekly conference, attended by all levels of the medical staff, in which dirty linen was aired. There were detailed discussions of errors of both omission and commission. The intent was not to embarrass or punish, but to learn from past mistakes. The medical service held a similar conference; at the MGH, it was called the "Allen Street" conference, named for the street used by hearses to access the morgue. Today, these are called "Mortality and Morbidity Conferences" and are required to be held with some frequency by all training programs. However, they are seldom weekly and almost never frank. They tend to be abstract, academic discussions of procedures or treatments rather than the particulars of recent errors. Each hospital has a "Risk Management" department that subtly (or not) influences the content of such exercises. "Risk Management" is an oxymoron; the "risk" at issue is not risk to the patient but risk for malpractice torts.

The ambience of the medical service was quite different from that of the surgical service. Students and interns (first-year residents) would round early on the patients they had admitted to the service in preparation for "work rounds." Work rounds assembled the students, interns, the charge nurse, one resident, and sometimes the attending. The ensemble moved from bed to bed. The intern and/or student who admitted the particular patient would present his or her status in detail, followed by the plans for the patient that day. The discussion that ensued was neither superficial nor imperious; options were aired openly, decisions made, and orders written. Customarily, the day started at 6:00 A.M. and work rounds finished around 9:30. There followed some thirty minutes to race around scheduling studies and other elements of busy work. From 10:00 A.M. till noon, the entire team (medical students, interns, the resident, and sometimes the nurses) would convene in a conference room for attending rounds. The new patients were presented by the student and/or intern who was admitting the day and night before. Then the group moved to the bedside, where a new patient was interviewed and examined by the attending. The group returned to the conference room to discuss the patient and his or her illness as thoroughly and comprehensively as possible. There were usually several newly admitted patients, and this format would be repeated for each. Only emergencies interrupted attending rounds; they were a sacred part of patient care. By noon, each patient was familiar to the entire team, both as an individual and as a clinical challenge.

Rounds ended and the work of the day commenced: new patients were admitted, either electively or through the Emergency Department; tests were ordered and results reviewed; consultations were requested and consultants engaged in discussions; discharges were planned; and families and patients engaged in conversations about status and course. It was a very busy undertaking before everyone could go home—everyone except the intern and medical student whose turn it was to stay overnight to care for the patients on the service and admit new patients presenting at all hours of the night. The pride of the inpatient service was the total immersion of all in the care of this group of patients. Learning curves for all were dramatic and did not involve just learning the tools and reflexes that made management efficient. There was a premium on comprehensiveness of care and understanding the patients' diseases. Literature was cited and discussed, and consultants were consulted for consultations, not just pronouncements. It was as physically demanding as life on the surgical services. It was also intellectually demanding, but in a context that was totally different from all that went before in preclinical education because of the immediate relevance to the circumstance of a particular patient. Many students would choose a career path that demanded less, but none would ever forget the intensity of the experience or denigrate its moral imperative.

In the early 1970s, teaching hospitals took pride in the rigor of their training programs. At the Massachusetts General Hospital, we worked in teams of two (one intern and one resident), alternating nights when we admitted patients. It took no time for most interns to learn the "ropes" of hospital routine. It also took no time for the intern to count on the experience the resident had gained in the year that separated them. And a symbiosis developed immediately: we knew each other and each other's patients and had no compunctions about helping the other with whatever was needed to care for the patient the other had admitted, nominally his patient (there was only one woman in my intern class, and none in the two classes ahead). The attendings were generally men of considerable clinical competence who kept the team grounded and thoughtful. Rotations on the medical service lasted a month each and occupied half the year; the remainder was largely for rotations on subspecialty services, which were mainly consultative. Nonetheless, working thirty-six hours out of every forty-eight for six months a year for two years was not for the faint of heart. While the MGH approach to training was legendary for its physical and intellectual rigor, sister elites matched it in their fashion. Essentially, we spent these formative years totally immersed in the goal of doing well by our inpatients. We developed reflexes and mind-sets that would advantage our patients throughout our careers.

Not every resident found the physical and emotional stresses of such intense training as exciting and meaningful as I did. Some found themselves overwhelmed—or a fish out of water. Several of the giants of twentieth-century medicine, including several in my cohort, moved on to other endeavors after the first year. But those of us who caught this wave have a bond to this day. By the time I became an attending at UNC in the mid-1970s, this model for clinical education had tempered. Generally, the two-doctor service had become a three-intern, one-resident service admitting every third night. But the drive to know the patient one admitted very well, and the patients one's colleagues admitted so well that there was no discontinuity of care when they were off duty, remained. So, too, did the rigor of work rounds and the intellectualism of attending rounds. I took the role of attending to heart. Nothing happened to the patients on our service without my cognizance, even if I made return visits to the bedside in the middle of the night. And I mastered the Socratic Method to a degree that few trainees will forget. "Where's the data?," no doubt, will be one of my epitaphs.

I mentioned that the charge nurse was part of the ensemble making work and attending rounds. That understates the way care was integrated in the inpatient service. The United States never adopted the British system, which placed the nurse ("sister") between the doctor and the patient. The United States applauded a partnership. Nurses truly participated in the morning rounding. Furthermore, every house officer going off duty would first round, yet again, with the nurses, who collaborated on problems and priorities; and the doctor on duty at night would round, yet again, with the nurses on the overnight shift for the same purpose. At least once a week, each intern would sit down with the charge nurse and review all orders in search of the redundant, the unnecessary, and the omitted. And at least once a week, each intern would meet formally with the social workers to discuss whatever contextual issues were pressing. Surgeons-in-training have long teased internists-in-training for their proclivity for endless rounding, and for good reason, but there is no better method to get to know the inpatients who are new to them and the institution, to care for and about them, and to foster career-long professionalism.

Evaluating clinical trainees in the 1970s and 1980s was a qualitative exercise. All had sat through myriad tests all their life. Clinical competence was left to peer review. In all my decades as a clinical teacher, I never ran into a major issue in peer review. The star student—the criteria for that moniker being related to performance at the bedside and during rounds—came along with some frequency, and the other students recognized it. All students were expected to be actively involved in the care of a limited number of patients with oversight by the resident, who in turn had oversight by the attending. The student presented the clinical history, examination, diagnosis, and therapeutic plan for the new patient on admission and updated during all subsequent rounds. Furthermore, the student did whatever needed to be done to carry out and modify the treatment plan. The student was a tightly observed member of the team. The resident had similar responsibilities for student patients and those without a student on the case. Performance was observed in real time, repeatedly, and in a very concentrated format. The inadequately performing trainee was easily recognized, although the approach to remediation was less well charted; it rarely led to dismissal. "Grading" was an exercise in peer review and a model for peer review going forward. Peer review may be an imperfect method for evaluating competence, but no alternative has been shown to be an improvement.

Teaching in the Clinic

American medicine in this era was in the process of differentiation. The primordial notion, dating back millennia, was that there were physicians and there were surgeons. By the 1970s, it was becoming less clear, and certainly less fashionable, to assume that each could maintain expertise across its purview. The surgeons took the lead in this with the argument that some technical prowess is exquisitely dependent on familiarity with particular diseases. In the 1950s, there were surgeons with HEENT on their shingle (Head Eyes Ears Nose and Throat); these differentiated into head and neck surgery, ophthalmology, and otolaryngology (ENT). Of course, there is further differentiation within each category, such as cornea and retina surgeons, but those lines remain a bit blurred. I suspect they will remain blurred because there are too few patients with unusual discrete diseases to support overspecialization. Otherwise, there would be specialists for the right nostril and specialists for the left. Nonetheless, many of the surgical subspecialties had evolved into discrete and independent specialties, such as gynecology and neurosurgery. In the academic world of the 1970s and 1980s, "surgery" still housed neurosurgery and orthopedics in many institutions. No longer.

However, "medicine" encompassed most of its subspecialties in the 1980s, with the exception of dermatology and neurology in some institutions. Today, the integration is very strained, but less so in the 1980s. All were internists; some were internists with specialized interests. And the subspecialization spoke more to intellectual focus than to technical competence. In the 1990s, cardiologists who worked in cardiac catheterization laboratories would be comfortable seeing patients with cardiac diseases who were not undergoing any procedures. For that matter, cardiologists were comfortable participating in the care of patients without heart disease. Today, there are "interventional cardiologists" who tend to tuck themselves into the catheterization laboratory the way radiologists stay in their radiology suites.

In the teaching hospitals, most specialists and subspecialists held clinics. Many of these were prominent physicians who were called upon to consult on cases in their sphere of expertise by physicians inside and outside the institution. Many would see such patients in follow-up over the long term. All of this was on a fee-for-service basis, compensating the academic department if the faculty was full-time salaried. I had such a rheumatology practice for over forty years in a teaching hospital clinic. The clinic in the usual teaching hospital of this era was a sparse facility built for function: small examining rooms; spare, often shared and sparsely furnished doctors' work areas; and waiting areas and "front desks" designed to be serviceable. The implicit message was that the patient and the doctor were to meet, hopefully with as little wait and fuss as possible; this was not a hotel. But this was a teaching hospital, and all patients came to expect exposure to a medical student or higher-level trainee, such as a resident rotating through the specialty or a "fellow" (post-residency training in the particular specialty is called a fellowship).

Teaching in the clinic was as varied as the proclivities, talents, and patient populations of the individual attending specialists. At one end of the educational spectrum was the attending who would delegate nearly all the consultation to a fellow or resident and, after hearing a summation, make a diagnostic or therapeutic pronouncement. Many such consultations were more than adequate from the perspective of the patient and the referring doctor. Furthermore, they offered exposures to the subspecialty discipline that advantaged the trainee as well. My own approach was at the other end of the spectrum. I managed to have two examining rooms in use simultaneously, and all my patients were thoroughly examined by a trainee working alone. Then I would enter the room with the trainee in rapt attention and repeat the entire examination, history, and physical examination. The trainees would learn what they had missed, if anything, and observe my approach to the patient. We then discussed the case, often with the patient's participation. It was real time education for all, including me and the patient. It was possible because of the leisurely pace of my clinic and the availability of two examining rooms. It is a teaching model that would no longer be supported by most institutions, including UNC Hospitals. The "pronouncement" model is more conducive to tight scheduling and "through put." I was not willing to compromise the leisurely pace and my lengthy give-and-take with the patient. It was the redundancy of the teaching method that was to be sacrificed to "through put" by subsequent iterations of the "teaching hospital."

Exporting the American Way

During the 1970s and 1980s, the era we are considering in this chapter, I was privileged to enjoy six semesters as a visiting professor at clinical institutions abroad. For each, I split my efforts between research and the clinical venue, with the latter always in an inpatient setting. Of these semesters, four were spent in a medical institution in London, one in Paris, and one in Kyoto Prefecture. I am not the first to observe the dramatic differences in the fashion in which medicine is taught and practiced across cultures. Of all who have written about this, few have done justice to the topic as successfully as the late Lynne Payer, who brought the perspective and observational skills of an investigative journalist to the task of contrasting the patient's experience in England, Germany, and France with that in the United States.[7] I'll settle for the particularly telling Japanese object lesson.

I was invited to participate in a demonstration teaching program in the municipal hospital in Maizuru, a small city in a beautiful setting north of Kyoto on the Sea of Japan. I initially demurred because medicine is grounded in illness narrative, and language skills are not my forte. But my host prevailed, granting a one-year delay for me to study Japanese and promising that I would have time to pursue my research interests in disability schemes. My host, Dr. Tadashi Matsumura, was the chief of medicine who had a dream and a mission. He was convinced that clinical education in Japan was sorely in need of major revamping. He had studied pulmonology in the United States for a year and was determined to bring the American approach to bedside teaching to Japan. He wanted his medical service to be the demonstration site and managed to make his intent so widely known that many Japanese resident physicians applied.

Before I describe the Japanese teaching service, you must realize that this was around 1990, when, by any measure, "health" in Japan was the best in the world, with longevity approaching the limits for our species. Furthermore, Japan had evolved a universal health-care system that was among the least costly in the industrialized world, a fraction of the American per capita expense even then. So whatever was going on in the Japanese health-care arena, it was not bad. But it was different. The pinnacle of the delivery system was the private-practice internist, who sees well over 100 patients per day and prescribes (and purveys) more pharmaceuticals per capita than anywhere else. The Japanese hospital and clinic buildings were dingy, most designed in the 1950s. And the average length of a hospital stay was three months. Patients were very compliant, families helped with nursing of their loved one, intensive care beds were few so that acute illnesses were treated in open wards next to convalescing patients, and patient-doctor communication was kept to a minimum. Remember that, despite all this, "health outcome" and cost-effectiveness were exemplary.

If the Japanese health-care system is not "broken," why would Dr. Matsumura want to "fix it," and how could I have the temerity to take on that charge? Good questions. Health, medicine, and the doctor-patient relationship are all socially constructed, meaning each reflects the preconceived notions of the participants. Culture is the product of these collaborations. Going to the doctor in France is a different experience from that in England, even though the "science" is shared. If the Japanese are long lived at little expense, why would we want to introduce elements of another culture that is not as successful by these criteria? The answer is socially constructed, too, and might well be described as chauvinism.

Japan has fully adopted and contributed to the evolution of modern science. What differs is the fashion in which medicine is practiced there. That has unique historical roots. The Tokugawa shogunate was able to largely isolate Japan from Western influences from 1641 to 1853, but not entirely. There was international trade, which introduced entrenched Western influences. In particular, the Netherlands was an established trading partner through the port of Nagasaki—so established that the port was home to an influential community of Dutch physicians. Hence, the Japanese approach to Western medicine was long comfortable with a highly patronizing form of the doctor-patient relationship. For a Japanese patient, or for that matter a Japanese student, to question the pronouncement of a "sensei" was simply anathema. One did what one was told, and did so promptly and efficiently.

Dr. Matsumura was bound and determined to establish a demonstration American-style teaching program in his Department of Medicine in the Maizuru Municipal Hospital, a community hospital. I was one of about a dozen American medical educators he recruited to the task, each staying a semester or more. Outstanding graduates of elite Japanese medical schools applied, all with some familiarity with English and some special drive to train differently—a drive derived from the stories of American education delivered by American films, media, and Japanese physicians returning from U.S. training stints. I and a dozen residents became "family" in this small municipal hospital, partaking in daily teaching rounds, journal clubs, mortality and morbidity conferences, and long discussions of the cultural differences in our approaches to caring for inpatients.

The American approach to attending and attending rounds was different, indeed, and for some it was far more appealing than Japan's approach. I saw that for myself when I was invited to serve as visiting professor on the rheumatology service at the teaching hospital of the elite Kyoto University medical school. More than a mountain range separated the Maizuru Municipal Hospital from the Kyoto teaching hospital in terms of national and international repute. But the physical facilities were not that different, and nor was the average length of stay. The service was staffed by a group of very bright, well-read residents who were very eager for an interactive learning experience. After all, the turnover of patients was very slow, so their education was not driven by the variability in clinical exposure. As is typical of a Japanese medical teaching service, attending rounds occurred once weekly and were quite perfunctory, usually involving a decree by the sensei as to the date for discharge. The trainees were largely on their own and impressively self-motivated. Furthermore, anything approaching a Socratic tradition is foreign to Japan's educational climate. Questioning and challenging are discomforting; I worked hard as an educator to create an environment where a student felt it appropriate to ask me why I said whatever I said.

Much has happened in Japanese medical education in the past couple of decades. It remains very hierarchical, termed "bunraku" for centuries. But many of the leading educators have followed Dr. Matsumura's lead in introducing a far more open and interactive intellectual climate. I wrote about the experience of teaching at the Japanese bedside in 1990,[8] concluding with the prophecy that before long, American teaching services will be recruiting Japanese educators to establish demonstration projects of the sort of teaching that once was the pride of American medicine and the envy of the world before we lost our way.

CHAPTER FOUR

The Assault on Clinical Education

The new millennium was to witness the end of the era of the American teaching hospital serving as the incubator for intellectualism at the bedside. The erosion of the clinical ethos that nurtured me and had become my passion occurred slowly, inexorably, and predictably.[1] Nonetheless, I found myself bewildered, but in the good company of other experienced clinical educators who enjoyed the respect of students and an extensive peer group but found themselves progressively disenfranchised in the academic health center. Many found themselves shifted to a nontenure "clinical" track. "Clinical professor" denoted a lesser station and lower value in the hierarchy than "professor." I remained a professor because of my "research productivity," a designation that was a euphemism for bringing research funding into the hopper regardless of the quality or content of the research. But I took pride in the fact that the clinical professors considered me their peer. We shared the pain of this time of transition.

We also shared an understanding of the limitations of our purview as educators. Yes, I "knew" the patients on the medical service when I was attending. But I never knew them to the degree I had come to know the patients in my referral clinic, patients who were contending with chronic rheumatic diseases like rheumatoid arthritis for decades. There is a reproach in this discrepancy. Teaching in the inpatient service at best addressed only a fraction of the experience of illness and none of the experience of health.

The goal of medicine is to facilitate, as much as possible, the transition from "patient" back to person. That requires knowing the person, or at least the person the patient aspired to be. For many, illness is both intermittent and remittent. For many others, returning to personhood requires the ability to compartmentalize persistent illness, to cope so well that one feels intact and valuable despite challenges that cannot be wholly avoided or avoided at all. I did not learn this in medical school or in my training years. I learned it when I first joined the faculty at UNC over forty years ago and a patient in clinic said, "Doc, I have a backache, and I don't know if I can go to work." That encounter opened my eyes to the fact that while diseases afflict organs, illness affects people. This patient was confronting what I came to call "the illness of work incapacity." I was so fascinated with the realization of the breadth of the illness experience that understanding and dissecting it superseded my work as a basic scientist to become the theme of my career as a clinical investigator.[2] More to the point, medicine misses the forest for the trees whenever it neglects the patient in the attempt to salve only the patient's disease.

Toward the end of the twentieth century, clinical education had been restricted to the inpatient to such an extent that medicine's humanistic tradition was sorely discounted. As a result, inpatients were underserved, the education of the next generation of physicians was skewed, and society at large was deluded into thinking that the "hospital" was a citadel that harbored all that was worthy in American medicine. Few in the academy realized this, and fewer cared. Most members of the faculty focused on their careers as investigators and considered their role as clinical educators to be ancillary. The clinical faculty was anxious but passive. Committed clinicians generally have nonconfrontational personalities and avoid conflicts. Notions of therapeutic relationships and clinical excellence were not completely silenced, just relegated to lower priorities in the minds of those responsible for feeding and watering the social construction of health in America.

And those who were responsible for the feeding and watering of this system of health care were gaining in number and in power. For them, medicine was never again to be seen as a cottage industry. Health care was never again to be seen as grounded in the patient-physician interchange. Medicine was not even to be seen as a profession or an institution. Medicine would be but one component of an industrial complex. Furthermore, it was already a major industry by any criteria, with impressive manpower needs, costliness, and administrative challenges. In the last decade of the twentieth century, the infrastructure supporting the care of the patient became the superstructure of an industry that commandeered an ever-inflating transfer of wealth. To that end, patients became units of care, diseases became product lines, and physicians became production workers.

This is the decade when all this evolution seemed sensible, and any argument to the contrary seemed irrelevant at best, if not contrarian, obstructionist, or obsolete. Nonetheless, the status quo was hardly defensible. One might try to defend what remained of the intellectualism of the teaching service, but little else about medicine would have escaped scathing criticism had it not been squelched. Furthermore, it seemed sensible that if intellectualism had to be sacrificed in order to nurture the hulking medical industry, so be it. And so it came to be.

Pinioning the Attending

Medicare subsidizes the training of physicians by allowing greater reimbursement for inpatient care in the teaching services.[3] The rationale is that the bed charges include money for the salary of resident physicians, just as for the salary of nurses. This mechanism does not provide support for fellowship training but is designed to provide a living wage for young physicians who are gaining more general skills and providing hands-on care in the process. How about the reimbursement of the attending faculty that are supervising the residents? Could they also receive a fee for their services? The Medicare program allowed for reimbursement of attending physicians' services if the "physician provides personal and identifiable direction to interns or residents who are participating in the care of his patient." As described in the prior chapter, this arrangement was loosely defined at the bedside, but not in the billing department. Attending on a teaching service generated a substantial portion of the departmental budget. But the degree to which the "physician provides personal and identifiable direction" escaped oversight. In 1980 Congress passed a law that was interpreted to require the attending "to exercise full, personal control over the management of the portion of the care for which payment is sought" and document such in the patient's chart. Most, including me, expected the medical student and/or resident to place a comprehensive daily note in each patient's chart. Most, including me, would round on the patients, review the note, amend it if necessary, and append a "Seen and agree" signature to the resident's or student's note. The relevant statute (IL-372) and HCFA (Health Care Financing Administration) were vague as to whether this was sufficient.

Some attendings were comfortable rolling up their sleeves and joining the interns and residents in a fashion that lent experience, wisdom, and presence to the immediate care of the patients. Other attendings lacked the skills and/or proclivity for such a role. Usually, they brought another contribution to the bedside, one that leaned heavily on their academic focus and often contributed substantially to the intellectual climate to which the team was exposed. For example, the attending might be expert in infectious diseases, even in the basic sciences that relate to infectious diseases, and was willing to share this expertise on rounds. In such a circumstance, the more senior of the residents stepped up and, along with consultants, provided the more practical input. Regardless of the fine details of the arrangement month-by-month, the integration of all levels of clinical expertise into the thinking and conversation at the bedside of each individual patient on a teaching service was the engine of the intellectualism that was the pride of American medical education. True, it was a pedagogical model that was wobbling on its pedestal because both teaching and clinical expertise were losing luster; they were increasingly seen as "loss leaders" in the financial model that was coming to dominate the academic health center. But the tradition of bedside rounding as more than an exercise in getting the work done was tolerated because of a Medicare fee schedule that supplemented bed charges to cover resident salaries and still paid the attending as the physician of record.

This cozy relationship came to a screeching halt in December 1995. HCFA and the U.S. Department of Justice decided that while these arrangements were defensible on educational grounds, they were a form of double-dipping. Medicare was reimbursing the hospital for the ministrations of the residents and also the attending physician for clinical activities that were redundant. Without admitting wrongdoing, the University of Pennsylvania settled a suit with the Department of Justice to pay almost $30 million in disputed billings and damages related to Medicare billing by attendings. The University of Virginia and other elite programs were similarly confronted, and all clinical teaching programs were sent scrambling.

A compromise between the Department of Justice and the medical schools resulted. The compromise is that if a medical school chooses to continue the traditional role, it could not bill separately for attending services. In order to bill, the attending must see every patient independent of the residents and document the examination in the chart in a detailed note that would be the basis for the billing. Medicare billing has been audited to this end ever since. I am not aware of a single medical school that was willing to lose the clinical income that attendings could generate. The business model of the modern academic health center depends on this clinical source of income. This seemingly mundane change in the finances of American clinical education led to a sea change in clinical pedagogy.

Every day, the attending physician has to independently see, examine, and document each new patient and then round independently on all others, again documenting in detail each patient's course and the attending's clinical plans. The physical burden on the attending approaches that of the three residents combined, although the attending is not required to personally place the order for tests, manage their scheduling, or the like. If an invasive procedure such as a spinal tap is done by a resident, the attending has to be present or immediately accessible in order to bill for the procedure. The tradition of the attending as an educator has been drastically curtailed. Few attendings can manage this workload for long; rotations are generally two weeks rather than four. Attending rounds are far less reflective, and notes by attendings and residents are designed to satisfy the auditors for billing purposes. It is rare to find a discussion that reveals the thinking process, and even rarer to find references to the clinical or scientific literatures in any chart in any American teaching hospital. (I know this because I have served as visiting professor in a great many of these hospitals.) There are ramifications for patient care that will occupy us in the next chapter. But there is a dramatic object lesson that provides a poignant preamble to those discussions.

Overworked

Libby Zion, a nineteen-year-old college freshman, died on March 5, 1984. She was a patient in a private room in New York Hospital, the elite, history-laden hospital in Manhattan that serves as the principal teaching hospital of Cornell Medical School. She had been admitted through the Emergency Department the evening before by Dr. Raymond Sherman, her family physician, for fluids and observation for a persistent "flu-like illness." As is typical of all teaching hospitals with private services, her care came under the wings of two house officers, Dr. Luise Weinstein (an intern) and Dr. Greg Stone (a first-year resident), who were also the house officers overseeing the care that night of many other private patients. They evaluated Zion and were puzzled as to the cause of her illness, particularly her "strange jerking movements." After consulting Dr. Sherman, they prescribed an opiate, Demerol, for sedation. Dr. Weinstein went about her business; Dr. Stone retired to an on-call room. Libby Zion did not do well. Her nurse informed Dr. Weinstein that Libby was becoming more agitated. Dr. Weinstein ordered restraints (leather belts that tied Libby down) and Haldol, a sedating major antipsychotic. That "calmed" the patient, but her temperature soared to 107 and she suffered a cardiac arrest. Efforts at resuscitation failed. The family was informed of her demise.

Libby's father was Sydney Zion, a Yale law graduate who went on to an illustrious career as a journalist and author. Mr. and Mrs. Zion's grief transitioned to anger as they became convinced that Libby had died because the care she received had been inadequate. Her doctors gave her Demerol, unaware she was taking a particular prescribed antidepressant, a combination that could lead to agitation and an uncommon catastrophic condition variously labeled "serotonin syndrome" or "neuroleptic malignant syndrome." These diagnoses can be distinguished by some biochemical features, but they share many clinical features, including high fever, neurological changes, and a propensity for cardiac instability. Both diagnoses call for discontinuation of the psychotropic agents and aggressive supportive care.[4] Rather than attempting to sort out Libby's downhill course, Dr. Weinstein ordered restraints and Haldol. Sydney Zion raged, "They gave her a drug that was destined to kill her, then ignored her except to tie her down like a dog." He called it "murder." In an op-ed in the *New York Times*, he wrote: "You don't need kindergarten to know that a resident working a 36-hour shift is in no condition to make any kind of judgment call—forget about life-and-death."

The Assault on Clinical Education

The "Libby Zion Case" became a tortuous legal battle. It commenced when the district attorney, Robert Morgenthau, considered an accusation of murder rather than malpractice, and it ended many years later when New York Hospital and the doctors were absolved in appellate proceedings. The legal transcripts are riddled with accusations in every direction and with a lot of devils in a lot of the details, so no clear lesson emerges regarding Ms. Zion's medical management, except that this was a great tragedy for all involved. One clear message that did emerge related to Sydney Zion's condemnation of the "36-hour shift." Committees were formed, meetings convened, professional organizations polled—all leading to recommendations by the New York State Department of Health in 1988 to restrict resident work hours.[5] The recommendation was that with the exception of the Emergency Department, individual residents who have direct patient care responsibilities shall not work on average more than eighty hours per week over a four-week period, or work for more than twenty-four consecutive hours. Furthermore, they should have one twenty-four-hour period off each week. The professional organizations raised issues about continuity of care and compromise in learning. Health economists raised issues about the cost of increasing the numbers of physicians to compensate for the decrease in coverage per doctor. But none of this was a match for the argument that patient care and safety was compromised if doctors were not sufficiently rested. The "Libby Zion Law" is Section 405 of the New York State Department of Health Code. In 1990 the Accreditation Council for Graduate Medical Education (ACGME) adopted similar regulations for all accredited internal medicine, dermatology, ophthalmology, and preventive medicine programs. In 2003 this regulation was expanded to all medical training programs in the United States, and in 2011 the ACGME restricted interns to sixteen-hour shifts.[6]

No one argues with the premise driving these regulations: exhausted physicians are more prone to mistakes than rested physicians. The arguments relate to whether patients are better served and residents better educated and trained as a result. The affirmative seems sensible. In Europe, it seemed so sensible that the corollary was accepted: restricting time at work would protect the health and safety of patients *and* the health and safety of trainees. It followed that restricting time at work should protect the health and safety of any worker, not just those involved in health care. In 1998 the Council of Europe in Brussels did just that: a directive was issued specifying minimum requirements for limiting exposure to the workplace for all workers. One mandate restricted all public employees to a forty-eight-hour workweek. This enormous social experiment was undertaken with no plans to monitor or measure its effectiveness. However, there have been attempts to assess the effect on resident education and on patient outcomes with observational data collected after the fact.[7] For example, about a dozen studies have been published attempting to measure the effect on resident education in the United Kingdom. Half of the studies inferred no effect and the other half a detriment. Observational data on patient outcomes such as in-hospital mortality, medical errors, and adverse events likewise discern little, if any, improvement. When 1,000 members of the Royal College of Surgeons were polled, 80 percent of consultants and 60 percent of trainees felt that care had deteriorated since the directive.[8] Of course, none of this is elegant science, nor does it speak to whether the directive affected the quality of patient care provided by physicians over the course of their careers if their training complied with the directive. Regardless, it is daunting to realize how disappointing the observational data have proved.

The directive may have seemed sensible to policy makers, but it never elicited approbation from European physicians and surgeons, nor were they surprised by the disappointing outcome data. They offer any number of explanations as to why the directive accomplished little if anything that was intended. In the UK, they point to the need to hire part-time and short-term ("locums") staff to cover when the full-time staff must be off duty. They point to the discontinuity of care and the hazards of communications between physicians and staff when responsibilities are passed off so frequently and often to staff with no prior exposure to the particular patient. For the surgeons, there is the added challenge of reduced operating time and unpredictable availability of supervision. Many practitioners found they could not adhere consistently to the directive according to their conscience. The president of the Royal College of Surgeons concluded that "to say the European Working Time Regulations has failed spectacularly would be a massive understatement."

The Assault on Clinical Education

The observational data and the debate in the United States are remarkably similar, even though the mandate is not for a forty-eight-hour workweek but an eighty-hour one. In the United States, rather than a proliferation of locums practitioners, the "night float" compromise took hold, and then the hospitalist movement. A "night float" is rotation where a resident is designated to step in for on-call residents after midnight, freeing up the on-call residents from additional admissions and helping out with patients already on the service so the on-call resident might catch a few winks. The job of the night float was to temporize as best they could until the primary treating doctors showed up in the morning, or, if temporizing was inadequate, put out clinical fires. The knowledge that night floats had about a particular patient was as comprehensive as the notes in the patient's chart. In the morning, the night float would "hand off" any new admissions to the team, review events that occurred overnight, and go home. Obviously, the "handoff" by the often exhausted "night float" is rife with the potential for lapses in communication that compromise continuity of care and increase the likelihood of medical errors.[9] Because of this, rather than revisit the issue of continuity of care, there are efforts to render handoffs more structured and comprehensive, perhaps making them more effective.[10]

The term "hospitalist" was coined in 1996 to denote physicians who are not residents but have completed training and are employed by the hospital to cover inpatient services when the primary treating physicians are off call, generally at night.[11] In essence, hospitalists are professional night floats. The nursing profession has evolved more along the "locums" model, with employment agencies that serve to market limited-contract nurses. I have met many a nurse who chooses this form of employment for its autonomy rather than contend with the nursing bureaucracies of the American hospital. A minority of full-time, inpatient registered nurses (RNs) actually nurse at the bedside, estimated at some 30 percent; the majority have administrative and supervisory positions. "Nursing" is more the job description of locums nurses and nurses with less training than is required for registration as an RN.

The specifics of the observational outcome data in the United States are no more encouraging than that generated in Europe. Since implementation of the 2011 ACGME duty-hour reform, there has been no significant change in thirty-day mortality rates or thirty-day readmission rates among Medicare beneficiaries in general, or among general surgery patients in particular.[12] In addition to all the observational data, there is even a randomized trial attempting to compare the effects of the ACGME 2011 sixteen-hour regulation with the less stringent 2003 version.[13] General medical teams were randomly assigned to three months on a schedule compliant with the 2003 regulation and then crossed over to three months on a schedule complaint with the 2011 regulation. The 2011 regulation-compliant schedule supported increased sleep duration for these teams when on call, but there was deterioration in educational opportunities and continuity of patient care. Furthermore, both the residents and nurses perceived an important decrease in quality of care—so important that the option of relying on a "night float" to comply with the 2011 regulation was discontinued.

Recently, directors of ACGME-accredited residency programs in internal medicine, surgery, and pediatrics were surveyed as to their impressions of the effectiveness of the 2011 regulations.[14] Of 730 eligible, 549 responded to the survey. Well over half felt that resident supervision, patient safety, the balance of service and education, scores on in-service examinations, and fatigue were unchanged by the 2011 regulations, not improved. More than half felt that the 2011 regulations had a negative effect on resident education, preparedness for senior roles, preparedness for primary responsibility for their patients, and continuity of care. Barely half felt that the quality of life for the residents was improved. However, the "price" was increased work for the directors and greater reliance on physician extenders such as nurse practitioners and physician assistants. There is also an increased burden on the more-senior residents, who find themselves rolling up their sleeves to provide care of patients left dangling by the more-junior residents, who can display "an almost frightening level of insistence on their new time and personal boundaries."[15]

The "Libby Zion Law" has provided residents with more time in the sack at the price of far less educational value to their training. The vaunted American teaching service of the twentieth century was lost by the millennium, one of the more dramatic unintended consequences of administrative wisdom that responded to the Libby Zion case. The price is not readily captured in "outcome" metrics in the observational data; patients are not worse off by the criteria that are readily measured. However, the most important asset of the vaunted American teaching service was its intellectual rigor and excitement. Absent these, the inpatient service is no longer an edifying way station in the course of life's trials and tribulations. Absent these, it's just a way station on a very potholed highway that is also traveled by the enforcers of regulations and highway robbers. And absent these, residency is a job that turns the acquisition of professionalism into a challenge, perhaps an insurmountable challenge.[16]

That brings us back to the saga of Libby Zion. Why did she die? Was she already developing the serotonin syndrome or the neuroleptic malignant syndrome on arrival at the Emergency Department? Possibly. But what followed were errors—errors that related to the incompleteness of her past medical history, particularly her history of prior drug exposures, followed by errors in judgment, in omission, and in commission on the part of her treating physicians. Would these errors have been obviated if there was a proactive ACGME at the time, and Dr. Weinstein, the resident on call, had a more leisurely workweek? Let's examine this line of reasoning closely.

It was 1984. The critical phase of Libby Zion's hospital course played out on the private pavilion of an elite teaching hospital. Her physician of record, her private physician, met her in the Emergency Department, evaluated her, discussed her with the two admitting residents, and went home. Libby was cared for by a nursing staff that was attentive; aware that she was doing poorly, they appropriately alerted the covering physicians, the residents rotating through the service at the time. That was Dr. Weinstein, an intern who was covering many other beds and responsible for any other private-service admissions that might come along that night. She responded with actions that were temporizing at best. That was what was expected of her in this clinical setting. The result was tragedy.

Libby Zion was admitted to a private service at New York Hospital by "covering" residents at the beck and call of her primary physician. This is an arrangement typical of private services in teaching hospitals at the time and many today. The role of the resident on the private service varied patient to patient depending on the practice style of their private physician. Some enjoyed a relationship that offered the resident as much responsibility as on a general medical service; the private physician served as the supervising and billing attending physician for his or her patient. If the private physician demanded exclusive control, the resident served more as a night float; if the circumstance demanded, the private doctor might be called and even called in, but the latter was unusual. The resident was called usually to temporize or even put out a fire. Libby Zion's resident temporized until the illness enflamed, and then it was too late.

One of the factors that cemented my decision to leave Massachusetts General Hospital and join the faculty of UNC and the staff of North Carolina Memorial Hospital forty-two years ago was a sign on the driveway that declared proudly, "Built By and For the People of North Carolina." North Carolina Memorial Hospital was digging its way out of its racist roots to offer to serve all the people equally. It never had a "private" pavilion. That appealed to me at the time. Of course, the thrust of this book is the historiography of the promise of "for the people"; tellingly, the sign disappeared from the hospital entrance to reappear as a tiny plaque hidden in the expansive marble lobby that is one of the many bland-modern structures that came to comprise UNC Hospitals and swallowed the original 1950s Georgian edifice in so doing. But in 1984, it was still the Georgian edifice, the North Carolina Memorial Hospital. I served as the attending physician on one of the general medical services about three months each year and always in July, when the new interns arrive bearing many more anxieties than clinical skills.

What would have happened if Libby Zion presented to the Emergency Department and was admitted to my service at North Carolina Memorial Hospital on that fateful night in 1984? There is no way for me to divine a different outcome. But I am certain of a different process. There were no designated Emergency Department physicians back then; internal medicine residents would have seen her and discussed her case with the internal medicine attending supervising them. If she had a private primary-care physician, he would have been called and consulted; there were very, very few private internists in Chapel Hill who had admitting privileges, and all were men. But while she was still in the Emergency Department, discussions would commence at her bedside. If she was confused in addition to feeling awful and twitchy, testing would commence. If she was also febrile, testing would have

The Assault on Clinical Education

been expedited. But if she seemed stable but puzzling, she would have been admitted to my service. The house officer on service that night would come to the Emergency Department with the medical student assigned to shadow and help. These two would examine Libby, confer, and confer with the Emergency Department internists. Many minds would have been brought to Libby Zion's bedside. If diagnostic uncertainty was deemed pressing, consultants would be called while still in the Emergency Department. If not, she would be transferred to a bed on my "service," which denotes both a particular medical team and a particular location in the hospital.

The resident on my service (there were no night floats yet, and the hospitalist movement was nascent) was physically on-site; even the on-call room was right there if a respite was feasible. And there were other residents covering neighboring services. If the duty nurse noted that Libby was deteriorating, the resident would be immediately available. Furthermore, when I was attending, my mandate was that I be called whenever the resident felt uncertain or insecure about any patient. I would have been called, and I would have been there promptly (my home is a mile away). A young woman who is "twitching," confused, and febrile would elicit a very aggressive diagnostic effort regarding metabolic abnormalities and infectious possibilities. Consultants would be mobilized even at night; in fact, there are designated specialty consultants for all the specialties in the hospital—usually a senior resident or fellow, and always with faculty backup on call. Furthermore, we would have a hair trigger regarding transfer into an intensive care bed. All this was possible in the teaching hospital of 1984 because that was what a teaching hospital in America was all about. Furthermore, we would be rushing to identify any treatable cause of Libby Zion's downfall and to support her physiology while doing so. I knew about "serotonin syndrome" and "neuroleptic malignant syndrome" in 1984, the latter mainly as a postoperative complication of anesthesia. I am not sure I would have recognized it out of that context then, though it was well described as an adverse effect of many drugs prescribed for psychiatric disorders, the serotonergic drugs.[17] There is no specific way to reverse the toxicity but many ways to support the patient while waiting, hopefully not in vain, for the syndrome to abate. Libby Zion would not have died restrained in a private room, nor would she have received Demerol or Haldol on an empirical basis.

I don't know New York Hospital today, let alone in 1984, except by reputation. It remains an elite teaching hospital. I suspect there were medical services similar to mine with clinical reflexes as finely honed to care for very sick patients in a teaching context. That means many examinations by residents and medical students and consultants. Libby Zion was not admitted to a teaching service, but to a "private service" where patient privacy and dignity were so sacrosanct that teaching was considered an intrusion. Libby Zion might well have died as quickly on a teaching service at New York Hospital, but she would have died surrounded by great intellectual fervor trying to postpone that fate.

Before you take away the notion that such intellectual fervor is exclusive to a teaching service, let me disabuse you. The American teaching services were largely quite effective; they taught two generations of physicians about the rigorous nature of caring for an ill inpatient. These students are the attending physicians in hospitals across the country, including nonteaching hospitals. Many (maybe most, but who knows) work in teams of attendings and nurses and are capable of mobilizing a great deal of intellectual fervor and diagnostic acumen for a patient such as Libby Zion—and they are willing to do so. These groups usually designate on-call physicians who are expected to function as I was on my teaching service: accessibly and willing to mobilize whatever was needed. Libby Zion died without such attempts because she was in a traditional "private" setting designed to limit the intrusive care that plagued patients on teaching services and not because of the "36-hour shift" condemned by her father. Her covering residents were constrained by tradition to temporize rather than take advantage of all that modern medicine can offer. Sadly, her treating doctors did not violate that "standard of care."

But no one in America appreciated that at the time, and few appreciate it to this day. To the contrary, the notion that a fatigued resident physician is a great threat to the well-being of the patient has become conventional wisdom. Sparing trainees from overwork remains a cause célèbre and a rallying cry of the movement to unionize residents. But it is a rallying cry that is missing the forest for the trees. Taking care of sick inpatients demands cooperation between all the professionals and allied health professionals involved. More than cooperation, it demands symbiosis. Part of learning to be a physician is learning one's limitations, as much in terms of clinical certainty as in terms of stamina. Every clinical setting that aspires for excellence in patient care must have mechanisms to provide assistance for its health-care professionals as expeditiously as is demanded by the clinical circumstance. Teaching hospitals and teaching services must model this behavior. It is the erosion of this modeling that we were witnessing with the pinioning of the attending and the focus on resident work schedules discussed above.

Errors

If anyone had any doubts that absentee attendings and exhausted residents were symptoms of the sad state of clinical education and the teaching hospital, they were soon dispelled. The nation was to learn that the American hospital in general, and the teaching hospital in particular, were dangerous to your health beyond the dangers of long and unsupervised work hours. In 2000 the National Academy of Sciences published "To Err Is Human: Building a Safer Health System."[18] This was the work of the Quality of Health Care in America Committee of the Institute of Medicine. The committee concluded that the nation had "an epidemic of medical errors," defined as "the failure of a planned action to be completed as intended or the use of a wrong plan to achieve an aim." The committee further estimated that "at least 44,000 people, and perhaps as many as 98,000 people, die in hospitals each year as a result of medical errors that could have been prevented." The nation was apprised and horrified. The American citadel of health care was not simply tarnished; it was pilloried. The report also concluded that most of these errors could be avoided by a "systems" approach—restructuring the processes involved in caring for patients that leads people to make mistakes and introducing processes that flagged errors before they were executed.

In a report a year later,[19] the committee detailed the changes in the system of health care that were necessary to effect a 50 percent reduction in these errors within five years. The report called for Congress to establish a Health Care Quality Innovation Fund of some $1 billion to "produce a public-domain portfolio of programs, tools, and technologies . . . and to help communicate the need for rapid and significant change throughout the health system." This funding had to wait for the "stimulus" legislation of the early days of the Obama administration. But many lesser projects were funded by many agencies, and the communication agenda escalated. Despite a decade of these efforts, the Office of Inspector General for the Department of Health and Human Services said in 2010 that adverse events contributed to the deaths of 180,000 Medicare-insured patients the previous year, and ten times as many suffered from a nonfatal adverse event.[20] By 2013 we were learning that preventable medical errors had climbed to the number-three cause of preventable deaths in America.[21] Something is very rotten in . . . our hospitals, or our calculations, or both. But the press, the public, and some policy wonks and researchers were convinced the problem only existed in the hospitals. This is a dialectic that precludes alternative explanations, including explanations that could promote patient safety.

The "quality" zealots hold sway to this day. But maybe they, like the "duty hours" zealots, continue to miss the forest for the trees. First, let's examine their definitions of avoidable errors more carefully. Some errors are clearly a reflection of the system of care gone awry. Operating on the wrong patient or the wrong knee, forgetting to remove surgical instruments from the abdomen, switching blood samples, administering medicines to the wrong patient, faulty equipment, and many more errors of this nature should be avoidable by improving the delivery system. In fact, thanks to the efforts of many in health policy and patient advocacy, great progress has been made. There are checklists in the operating room, redundant labeling systems, and much more that should have greatly reduced the possibility of human errors of this nature with technological solutions. But progress has been slow. Between 2005 and 2011, the adverse-event rates in American hospitals did not decline for surgical patients or patients with pneumonia, only for patients with cardiac conditions.[22] More specifically, the implementation of surgical safety checklists into the hospitals of Ontario, Canada, was not associated with a reduction in operative mortality or complications.[23] Lucian Leape is one of the most influential of those advocating for improving the quality of care and a principal voice in the National Academy's "To Err Is Human" polemic for a "systems" approach. He is inclined to dismiss these disappointing observations on the basis that they did not exclude the possibility of various forms of noncompliance.[24] Perhaps he is correct. However, adjusting for the magnitude of the procedures and for the severity of the illnesses of the patients, operative mortality and thirty-day postoperative mortality in acute-care hospitals was less than 1 percent, with or without a checklist. Furthermore, all surgical complications, fatal or nonfatal, afflicted less than 4 percent of patients. These are not trivial numbers, nor are they alarming, as they are likely to reflect the degree of desperation that drove the decision to operate in the first place. Routine procedures in well patients, such as hernia repairs or breast biopsies, do not carry anywhere near this risk.

Errors in process, obvious errors such as giving the wrong dose or leaving a sponge in the abdomen—all of which are incontrovertibly errors—are not the preponderance of preventable medical errors in general and preventable fatal medical errors in particular. Most of the fatal errors that led to the horrifying statistics that elicited national outrage were judgment calls, defined as errors either by peers reviewing medical records or by virtue of the voluntary reporting of errors by doctors and hospitals. Not long after the National Academies published "To Err Is Human," a study from the U.S. Veterans Administration demonstrated that the preventability of hospital deaths due to medical errors was very much "in the eye of the reviewer."[25] A panel of fourteen board-certified, trained internists undertook multiple structured reviews of the records of 111 hospital deaths, accumulating 383 reviews. They were measuring whether the deaths were "preventable by better care." About a quarter of the deaths were rated as possibly preventable by optimal care. However, a tiny minority would have left the hospital alive had optimal care been provided. The reviewing clinicians estimated that only 0.5 percent of patients who died would have lived three months or more in good cognitive health if care had been optimal, representing one patient in 10,000 admissions to the study hospitals. In-hospital deaths are largely the fate of very ill patients suffering from diseases in the terminal phases, or suffering from multiple confounding conditions simultaneously, or the frail elderly. Many of these patients die in Intensive Care Units where much is happening to them quickly, often under the pall of desperation, and where errors are usually apparent in retrospect rather than in the heat of the moment.

There's the Forest

The specter of avoidable complications, including avoidable deaths, has permeated notions of health-care reform for twenty-five years. Blame has been spread thickly and widely under the rubric "human error." Solutions have come in a torrent of regulations aimed at improving human performance. Some have proved ineffective if not counterproductive, such as restricting trainee hours, which has fragmented care and toned down intellectual rigor. In the torrent of regulations are attempts to supplant human performance with computerized algorithms—with consequences that were both intended and unintended, which will occupy us in chapter 7.

The emphasis of the "error" in human error is readily defensible, though the notion that "error" is an epidemic is indefensible. Even more indefensible is the fashion in which emphasizing "error" has come to deemphasize the "human" of human error. Several of my earlier books speak to the harms of medicalizing predicaments of life, an emphasis that would call into question our proclivity to screen and forewarn when we can't demonstrate a salutary outcome from the screening and forewarning. These heavily referenced books also discuss "Type 2 Medical Malpractice," which is the doing of the unnecessary, even if it is done well. I argue that such overtreatment is a medical error that is a scourge flying under the radar of health-care reform.

The American way of dying in a hospital is yet another instance of Type 2 Medical Malpractice. This is the setting where most "errors" occur, errors of commission in the desperate attempt to "save" the lives of the elderly, the frail, and the terminally ill. The message that merits wide debate is whether this is an appropriate way to die in America. My colleagues estimate that at least 40 percent of the patients in our many Intensive Care Unit beds at any given time have terminal illnesses. The best we can do with "optimal care" is to prolong their dying. The other 60 percent may benefit from all the hustle, bustle, and hassle of intensivists' medicine, perhaps in part because their biology is more forgiving of occasional "suboptimal" care that eludes the checklists and other systems safeguards.

America has made a tremendous investment in Intensive Care Units. We have many times the ICU beds per capita as any other resource-advantaged country: twenty-five per 100,000 people, as compared to five per 100,000 in the United Kingdom. Not surprisingly, when we build them, we also build the demand—so-called demand elasticity.[26] The indications for admission to these units in America result in a very different case mix than anywhere else. We need ICU beds for the likes of a Libby Zion and many others with acute or potentially reversible conditions, but do we need them for the frail elderly or the terminally ill? Maybe the error is not so much in their medical treatments as in the lack of appreciation of their humanity.

Sacrificing the Patient on the Altar of Industrialization

"Blaming the victim" for being too ill or too frail is not to excuse the preventable fatal medical error. Nor is it to excuse the incident non-fatal error that caused harm or could have done so. There are great efforts to raise institutional awareness of safety issues, the "safety climate of an organization," but the safety climate has proved as difficult to measure as the benefits of raising it.[1] Nonfatal adverse events are even more in the eye of the beholder than fatal events; differences in definition and in measurement can result in a tenfold difference in incidence.[2] Many scholars have bent their shoulders to this wheel and continue to do so. (The April 2011 issue of *Health Affairs* is dedicated to these efforts and provides a nice overview.)

It is politically incorrect if not reprehensible to do other than applaud all this effort. I do not think it unprincipled in the least. I do, however, think the approach is so slanted that it misses the mark. I am an inveterate advocate for the safety of each patient and for the provision of optimal care for each patient, one at a time. The current approach to quality and safety is anchored in the "systems approach" first advocated by Lucien Leape and reiterated in "To Err Is Human." This is an approach that borrows heavily from the work of W. Edwards Deming and later Bill Smith. Deming (1900–1993) was an engineer who earned a Ph.D. in physics at Yale. The aftermath of World War II found him on General Douglas MacArthur's staff offering lessons in statistical process control to Japanese business leaders. He continued to do so as a consultant for much of his later life and is considered the genius behind the Japanese industrial resurgence. The principle underlying Deming's approach is that focusing on quality increases productivity and thereby reduces cost; focusing on cost does the opposite. Bill Smith was also an engineer who honed this approach for Motorola Corporation with a methodology he introduced in 1987. The principle of Smith's "six sigma" approach is that all aspects of production, even output, could be reduced to quantifiable data, allowing the manufacturer to have complete control of the process. Such control allows for collective effort and teamwork to achieve the quality goals. These landmark achievements in industrial engineering have been widely adopted in industry, having been championed by giants such as Jack Welch of General Electric. No doubt they can result in improvement in the quality and profitability of myriad products, from jet engines to cell phones. Every product is the same, every product is well designed and built, and every product is profitable.

If patients were widgets, if caregivers were production workers, and if caring conformed to "six sigma" principles, errors would be easy to recognize, those responsible for the failures could be singled out for improvement, and remedies would be obvious. But manufacturing cell phones has little in common with managing the care of patients in all their variability and with all their unpredictability. No clinical metric conforms to a six sigma standard; we in medicine are comfortable defining "normal" with a 95 percent confidence interval, and we are fully aware that "outliers" can be clinically normal and those in the normal range abnormal.

Whereas many of the health-policy wonks speak of "six sigma" as if it came down from Mount Sinai, Deming appreciated the limitations early on and wrote/lectured widely about the various provisos. He prescribed little in the way of systems methodology, except making changes incrementally and testing each version scientifically (the Deming/Shewhart cycles). Deming understood the organic nature of any industrial process. He placed great value on what he called "profound knowledge": the laws of variation, the theory of knowledge, the theory of systems, and psychology. I have no doubt that Deming would find the direction America is taking with health-care policy doomed from the outset. One of my oldest friends, a college roommate, is Brooks Carder, Ph.D. Brooks is a leading industrial psychologist with a very interesting career path. He is a disciple of "The Compleat Deming" and has written extensively about the implications of his legacy.[3] No doubt Deming's "profound knowledge" would not just take into account the variability that is inherent in the care of patients; it would celebrate the unpredictability of the human predicament.

It is hard for me to imagine that others have not come to grips with this realization. But it certainly doesn't seem so from the federal policy agenda, the regulatory climate, and the burgeoning industry that has grown to service the quality agenda. Suffice it to say that mandating record keeping designed to create data sets with the "granularity" to monitor process and outcomes is an enormous and enormously expensive undertaking as well as a fool's errand. But the industry servicing this errand is but one of the new initiatives involved in the quality agenda. There are various "teamwork" initiatives, such as Accountable Care Organizations (ACOs), that are subsidized. There are carrot-and-stick initiatives that compensate more generously if doctors can demonstrate they are adherent with practice and reporting guidelines put forth by Medicare and other insurance companies, a form of "pay-for-performance" initiative. There is another industry that informs these guidelines. Small advocacy groups have grown into sizable, influential organizations, such as the National Quality Forum (NQF) and the Institute for Healthcare Improvement (IHI), which employ more than 100 senior staff members to capture and disburse the many millions of dollars procured from governmental and private sources. For example, NQF receives $10 million annually to provide CMS (the Medicare administration) the performance measures it uses to measure the quality of the treatments it purchases. NQF generates these measures by a consensus process that it purports to be transparent and free of overt bias.

All this effort should invoke the "profound knowledge" that Deming knew was necessary to render notions of "quality" ethical. Sadly, there is as much room in this effort for conflicts of interest to rear an ugly head as in many other aspects of medical practice.[4] Some are more than scandalous; they are dramatic object lessons. For example, NQF has been faced with such scandals. Dr. Charles Denham was dismissed from chairing an NQF committee charged with establishing certain performance measures after the Department of Justice accused him of profiting from kickbacks to the tune of $11.6 million. Denham claimed he had legitimate contracts with the drug company that profited handsomely from the performance measures his committee established. Maybe so, but that does not absolve him, since he had not recused himself or even declared his financial connections while his committee put forth self-serving recommendations. Obviously, "pay-for-performance" must be driven by the patient outcome that results from the performance rather than its profitability. That's why an exposé by ProPublica (February 12, 2014) has raised eyebrows. Christine Cassel is a very distinguished internist who has written extensively about ethical issues in medicine. She was appointed president and CEO of NQF in 2012 after serving as president and CEO the American Board of Internal Medicine for a decade. It turns out that in 2013, she was paid hundreds of thousands of dollars by two large medical companies that have a stake in NQF's work. She was paid about $235,000 in compensation and stock as a board member for Premier, Inc., a Charlotte, North Carolina, company that says it provides group purchasing and performance-improvement consulting for an alliance of 2,900 hospitals and thousands of nursing facilities and other providers. She had also been paid nearly as much for several years as a board member for the Kaiser Foundation Health Plans and Hospitals. Whether such relationships represented conflicts of interest in her role with the American Board of Internal Medicine is debatable. However, few would argue that point regarding her role at NQF. What was she thinking when she accepted the position at NQF without first divesting herself of all potential conflictual relationships? Helen Darling, who is the chair of the board of directors of NQF (and president of the National Business Group on Health), told ProPublica that the board was "fully aware" of Dr. Cassel's outside board service. Dr. Cassel has since divested. What were they thinking when they recruited Dr. Cassel?

There are a number of other people, similarly prominent participants in the health-policy tableaux, who tend to discount the implication of associations such as those Dr. Cassel maintained with interested stakeholders. They seem to feel that such remunerative relationships are not proof of bias, not even an indication of the likelihood of bias.[5] Shouldn't a physician of Dr. Cassel's repute be able to rise above such influences and offer her expertise to the NQF and to Premier, Inc., evenhandedly? Perhaps, but I lean toward Rosemary Gibson's opinion, which was paraphrased in the ProPublica report: so much money permeates decision making in Washington, she said, that participants have become oblivious. "The insiders don't see it," Gibson said. "It's like a fish in water." Gibson, whose highest degree is a master's from the London School of Economics, has long been embroiled in issues that relate to the ethical boundaries of health care. She is a senior advisor to the Hastings Center, an influential, not-for-profit, freestanding think tank focused on bioethics. She spearheaded the Robert Wood Johnson Foundation's health-care quality program for years. She is a public director of the ACGME. And she wrote the influential book *Wall of Silence*, which puts a human face on the deliberations that led to the Institute of Medicine's report "To Err Is Human."

Gibson's reflection brings to mind the tremendous debates and occasional scandals regarding conflictual relations that embroil many "guideline" and "advisory" panels that were constituted to serve the needs of patients who are the constituency of advocacy organizations (such as the American Heart Association and the American Cancer Society) or federal agencies (such as the Food and Drug Administration). Unfortunately, object lessons continue to appear. British guidelines for treating the acute heart attack and American guidelines for reducing blood lipids seem straightforward and sensible, but they are not. They both suffer from conflicts of interest, the former from peer pressures and preconceptions[6] and the latter from financial shenanigans.[7]

Conflictual relationships plague nearly every aspect of the health-care system, including the leadership of the educational establishment. In the spring of 2014, a commentary was published in the *Journal of the American Medical Association* titled "Conflict of Interest Policies for Academic Health System Leaders Who Work with Outside Corporations."[8] In their essay, Etta Pisano, Robert Golden, and Laura Schweitzer argue that "leaders have a responsibility to set an example for others in their institution, especially for those training to be health care professionals." When the article was written, Etta Pisano was dean of the College of Medicine at the Medical University of South Carolina in Charleston and Bob Golden was dean of the School of Medicine at the University of Wisconsin in Madison. Both earned their academic and administrative spurs as my colleagues on the faculty of the University of North Carolina, Etta in radiology and Bob in psychiatry. Bob has had influential roles in organizational psychiatry, but I never knew him to be entangled with corporate entities. Etta, on the other hand, must have been writing from the perspective of someone who had an epiphany. Her claim to fame was as a proponent of digital mammography. Etta's work and advocacy were very much intertwined with the marketing agenda of the General Electric Corporation, the leading manufacturer of the necessary hardware. Furthermore, she was one of myriad assistant and associate deans working for the chief executive officer/dean of the medical school, a man who was compensated for sitting on the board of Medco at a time when Medco was the pharmacy benefits manager for the North Carolina state health plan.

The heated rivalry between UNC and Duke University does not play out solely in the athletic arena. Dr. Victor Dzau resigned as Duke's chief dean and executive in the summer of 2014 to assume the role of president of the Institute of Medicine. That appointment was met with controversy regarding Dr. Dzau's positions on the boards of PepsiCo, Medtronic, and other companies that have products that relate to "health" and "health care."[9] These are lucrative positions that supplement his salary from Duke's not-for-profit health system, a salary that was listed as $2.8 million in 2012. Furthermore, he had accumulated a sizeable stock portfolio in companies for which he served as a director. He divested himself of some, maybe all, of these unseemly relationships once the issue was raised. Maybe Etta Pisano has had an epiphany, but is it too little, too late?

Conflictual relationships aside, despite multiple attempts of varying scope and quality, none of these "quality" initiatives have been shown to result in meaningful improvements in clinical outcomes or a meaningful decrease in adverse events. Rather, as with the assault on resident work hours, they are effete at best and often counterproductive. Maybe the innovation that NQF and IHI promise to find and fund is out there, eagerly awaiting discovery. Maybe not; maybe the "quality" effort has been seduced by a systems approach that only advantages manufacturing industries and similar stakeholders. Maybe the assumption that health care is an industrial enterprise is a sophism. Regardless, the entire effort is a pall over the clinical arena. It is yet another layer of obstruction placed between a patient seeking rational caring and a doctor who wants to provide it.

Byzantium

For the sake of safety, inpatient care in the teaching hospital has been fragmented. In response to fiscal contingencies at CMS (the

Medicare/Medicaid administration center), teaching on the "teaching" service has been pruned. Furthermore, under the banner of cost savings, the duration of inpatient stay has been made a basis for reimbursement, so that patients must have a problem for which admission to a hospital is deemed indemnified by an outside agency rather than deemed appropriate or necessary by the patient and the doctor, and there must be a treatment plan that is focused on that problem. Everything else is to be dealt with outside the hospital, or downplayed, or even ignored. Everything else includes confounding illnesses, incidental findings, and the patient's challenges in coping. Everything else includes teaching, discussions of uncertainty, consideration of alternative approaches, mentoring in peer relationships, discussions of the many ethical contingencies that surround much of patient care, and all else that was the pride of the vaunted American teaching hospital when it was still vaunted. The pressure is for discharge from the moment of admission. Reimbursement depends on it.

This is a pressure that demands an ever-more-efficient elimination of "everything else." That pressure has nearly banished the internist and the general medical service from the American teaching hospital. In its place are myriad specialty services. After all, if you have a kidney problem, it makes sense that the "renal team" could focus on it best, and the renal service could be designed to handle kidney problems. If the renal service patient has an urgent nonrenal issue, consults can be called. If it's less urgent, it can be managed after discharge. The arrangement probably decreases inpatient time significantly. It definitely deprives the patient, the students, the residents, and even the renal attending of informative discussions beyond the specifics of nephrology, the medical specialty that focuses on kidney disease. The specialists grow more and more narrow in their intellectual scope and model such narrowness for all they are mentoring.

Of course, some of this efficiency is readily justified, usually on technological grounds. Surgical patients should be admitted to a surgical service because the staff there is comfortable with the care of the surgical wound and postoperative complications. Surgical patients might be a fish out of water on a medical service. Even the medical services, like the renal service, have a technological rationale as the staff becomes familiar with the challenges of patients on renal dialysis. However, there is much about kidney disease itself that merits open discussion—and much about kidney disease patients that does not relate to their kidney disease, since kidney involvement is a manifestation of many other diseases that target more than the kidney, such as lupus and diabetes. In the teaching services of yore, students, residents, and consultants crossed all these barriers in engaging in discussions and debates about alternative diagnoses and treatments. No one has the time for such interactions anymore; the only focus is on what is necessary to hasten discharge. Sadly, fewer and fewer realize what the patients, students, residents, and consultants are missing out on.

Of course, this carries over into the clinics. More and more, specialty clinics are physically freestanding. The business model countenances multiple buildings scattered about the community to capture the trade. The notion that "everything else" will be dealt with as an outpatient is tarnished at best. When consultants worked side-by-side, informal "curbside" consultations were commonplace: "Hey, Joe, got a minute to look at this patient with me?" We all had a minute, and we all never abused one another because what goes around comes around. For years, I saw "rheumatology" patients in facilities that housed multiple specialists. No longer is a curbside consultation the rule (and administration is happier for it since it was never billed). In fact, seldom is a curbside consultation even possible; the consultant likely is in another building. Of course, this means inconvenience and delay for the patients, often considerable delay depending on the consultant's schedule (mine is measured in months). It also means a dearth of intellectual cross-fertilization and a narrow experience for the trainees.

All this has come to pass for the sake of the business model. But the business model has an impressive growth curve and insatiable avarice. Attendings, consultants, residents, fellows, and patients are simply fodder.

Invasion of the Trialists

Speaking of avarice, the pharmaceutical industry and the corporate medical center were a marriage made for Dante's Inferno. There are lengthy discussions of the potential for and reality of conflictual relationships between physicians and the pharmaceutical and medical-device industries in several of my earlier books. I also cite the data that document the degree to which industry contributes to the "educational" budgets of medical schools and their constituent departments, contributions that have no contractual strings attached. In 2007 over two-thirds of department chairs and over two-thirds of departmental administrative units had financial relationships with pharmaceutical companies or other for-profit health-care stakeholders.[10] There has been a great deal of discussion of these relationships and some modulation, including push-backs and restrictions. The efforts to mitigate if not eliminate the potential for bias that conflictual relationships bring to medical education at all levels are ongoing and concerted.[11]

However, when so much money is at stake for so many stakeholders, innovative approaches to the creation of conflictual relationships are predictable—and there are many. Some that have infected the educational climate are still sailing below the radar. One hides under the rubric of "translational research." This is a neologism that is designed to ring beneficent. We have an enormous amount of interesting new science bubbling out of myriad laboratories around the world, science that informs a range of disciplines, from genomics and proteomics to designer drugs and so much more. Short of testing hypotheses in volunteers, there is no way to know if any of the fruit of this new science is clinically meaningful rather than solely intrinsically interesting. Animal studies are of limited utility; there are many examples of toxicities that are only apparent in our species and many more of efficacies that are species specific. At some point, human testing is necessary. This is "translational research," translating from the laboratory to the patient.

The algorithm for translational research is well established and closely monitored by the Food and Drug Administration (FDA). It should be an elegant and ethical undertaking that sorts the wheat from the chaff. But it has been distorted to serve agendas other than the sorting. It is rare that studies are designed with the expectation that a new drug or an old drug with a new indication will be dramatically efficacious. Most translational research is designed to seek small effects. The smaller the effect, the larger the study population needed to discern the effect. Take the example of a drug you expect to work in one patient out of 200. If you compare the outcomes in 200 patients given the drug with the outcomes in 200 patients given a placebo, it is likely you will not discern any benefit. You have to run the numbers of subjects up into the thousands or even tens of thousands to stand a chance of discerning a difference in outcome between those on the drug and those on the placebo. Hence, "translational research" is an enormous enterprise that requires multiple research sites, each recruiting gaggles of volunteers. It is such an enormous enterprise that it spawned an entire industry, contracted research organizations (CROs), that take over the entire process all the way to data analysis, the presentation of results, and the preparation of new drug applications to the FDA. The CROs are paid by the pharmaceutical industry to recruit subjects or to pay physicians to do the recruiting. The CROs also are funded to pay for the mechanics of the study, including paying physicians to recruit subjects ("finders' fees") and for carrying out the study.

Much wealth is transferred under the banner of "translational research." Some of the CROs are large, profitable, publicly traded corporations such as Quintiles Transnational and PPD. But many established medical organizations, from multispecialty clinics to academic health centers, have realized that there is gold to be mined in "translational research." Most academic hospitals have, or are trying to develop, their own CROs; some are sizable undertakings, such as at Duke University Medical Center, and others aspire to compete. Most of the "translational research" in academic centers is collaborative, functioning as one of the participating centers studying a particular drug. The gold ring goes to the organizing center that receives the lion's share of the money. The result is that the clinical academy has grown a new breed of physician, the trialists, and a new source of income, the CRO, both of which have presence in the intellectual community—often considerable presence.

So far, nothing seems disconcerting. But the devil is in the details yet again. Seeking small effects in large trials serves the business model of the pharmaceutical industry much more reliably than it serves any patient. Some of these trials are simply "seed trials." These are marketing exercises masquerading as attempts to find new indications, new combinations, or new dosing of drugs that are already licensed. They are designed to familiarize the trialists with the agent with the expectation that the trialists will serve as "thought leaders" and influence their communities. This scheme works. Furthermore, trialists are often on formulary committees that determine the drugs that hospitals stock in their pharmacies. All this creates the heuristic that physicians and trainees carry forward to the bedside of their patients in the future.

But there's an even more insidious downside to large trials seeking small effects. First of all, one needs to ask up front whether a small effect is clinically meaningful. If you need to treat 20 patients for some period of time to benefit 1 patient (an NNT, or "Number Needed to Treat," of 20), would you take the agent yourself? Perhaps, but the decision would be colored by the magnitude of benefit, the likelihood of adverse events, and the out-of-pocket costs. It is not a foregone decision. How about an NNT of 50, or 200, or more? Soon the negative decision is foregone.

Distorting the Notion of a Clinically Meaningful Benefit

If the most benefit one could hope for is either so trivial or so unlikely to be a rational choice, why is the intervention subjected to "translational research"? The answer lies in the evolution of licensure by the FDA. The 1962 Kefauver-Harris Amendments to the Food, Drug and Cosmetic Act stipulated a demonstration of efficacy as prerequisite to licensure of any pharmaceutical. At the time, biostatistics was still in its infancy. The efficacy mandate has fueled that field's dramatic growth and its dominance of the decision for licensure. Very rapidly, the notion of "statistical significance" became more than a minimal requirement for licensure; it became the requirement. Results of the "Phase 3" randomized controlled trial (RCT) became determinative. Was the difference in outcome from exposure to the active agent compared to the referent agent (usually a placebo, sometimes a standard therapy) no more likely to occur by chance alone 5 times out of 100? This is statistical significance, usually expressed as a probability; for example, it would not happen more than 5 percent of the time by chance alone ($p < 0.05$). This is a convention based on a gambler's mindset. If you are a high-risk gambler, you might be willing to swallow the agent even if it was more likely to be no better than a placebo. But convention demands that the agent be shown to be better than placebo in a Phase 3 RCT with a $p < 0.05$.

For a clinician, the patient, and the patient-doctor collaboration, this is inadequate information upon which to base a decision. What is the benefit of an outcome that wouldn't happen more than 1 time in 20 tries by chance alone? Maybe the statistically significant benefit sounds impressive, such as a 50 percent increased likelihood of survival. But a gambler would immediately know that such an assertion is inadequate information to make a decision. If 3 of 1,000 patients with a lethal disease survive a year on the drug, and only 2 who don't take the drug survive a year, would you take the drug? Do you believe that such an infrequent event can be measured reliably and reproducibly? Wouldn't it seem reasonable to take a chance on your being an "outlier" without the drug, particularly if there is any downside to taking the drug (adverse effects, co-pay, etc.). That would be like winning the lottery without buying a ticket.

These considerations of clinical significance are not as determinative at the FDA as the statistical significance. Perhaps the financing of the FDA has something to do with this emphasis. FDA determinations are underwritten in part by fees charged to the company submitting the application for licensure. This is an inherently conflictual relationship.

Speaking of inherently conflictual relationships, let's reconsider the CRO. The philosophy of science since David Hume calls for a refutationist perspective, a perspective elaborated on by John Stuart Mill and further developed by Karl Popper. Science is a process by which any hypothesis is tested by challenging its validity. "Truth" is the hypothesis yet to be disproved. "Truth" is always tentative. But subliminally, if not overtly, a pharmaceutical firm does not give a CRO tens of millions of dollars hoping that the drug will prove ineffective. Furthermore, drug trials looking for small effects require large populations of subjects and are always "sloppy," with missing data points, dropouts, subjects who take other drugs, and the like. An unencumbered scientist does her level best to analyze such data predisposing the analysis toward lack of benefit. Conversely, CROs are encumbered by the charge to serve their client well enough that the client will return with another contract. There are many examples of industry-sponsored trials that are plagued by prejudicial data, sometimes to the extent of being criminal activities, even in CROs based in medical schools.

All this is a plague on clinical decision making. The FDA is primed to license agents that can't be shown to have more than marginal efficacy. The CROs are primed to massage data seeking statistically significant yet clinically insignificant outcomes. The pharmacy is awash in such agents and their "me too" competition. All of this spills over into the clinical arena that is nurturing the next generation of physicians.

The clinical literature is dripping Phase 3 trials. Some are in the most influential of medical journals, often next to full-page advertisements by pharmaceutical and device firms for the same agents that are described in the scientific articles. There are so many trials, including so many on the same or similar agents, that the clinical literature is also dripping review articles, even systematic review articles that attempt to merge the inconsistent outcomes in these trials in quest of a greater truth. There is a formal methodology for doing such, a meta-analysis, although it too has a good deal of room for judgments as to which of the inconsistent trials should be relied on more than others. There are even organizations, often with overt vested interests, publishing meta-analyses. It is no surprise that trials that are industry sponsored and meta-analyses that are industry sponsored are more likely to favor the particular agent than trials or meta-analyses sponsored by governments.

Furthermore, remember our example of the 50 percent reduction in mortality that sounded seductive until one probed the details and learned that the benefit was trivial and likely to be unreliable? The 50 percent number is a *relative* risk reduction; the 1 in a 1,000 is the *absolute* risk reduction. Everyone agrees that no journal article or advertisement should shout out the former without shouting out the latter even louder. Nearly everyone who agrees is aware that this mandate is consistently violated. That prejudices the decision making, not only by the patient but also by the doctor. It requires familiarity with the details of the data and time to explain this exercise in marketing to the patient. As I've long said, it takes twenty seconds to write a prescription in America and twenty minutes not to.

Perhaps the most disquieting aspect of this narrative relates to surgical devices and procedures. These are licensed as long as the practitioners/purveyors exclaim benefit and can document that there is nothing new about their offerings in terms of materials that might be harmful. No Phase 3 RCT efficacy trial is a prerequisite to licensing. Furthermore, while "detail" salesmen from the pharmaceutical industry are now banned from most academic health centers, their counterparts in the device/procedure world are welcomed for their ability to instruct the practitioners on the nuances of the application of their devices. Many are credentialed so that they can accompany surgeons into the operating room. Of course, many a surgeon has a vested interest in the particular devices and is a more-than-willing host.

To my eye, the "stakeholders" have commandeered the academic health centers. They contribute mightily to the budget of the center and the individual components. They have managed to recruit many a "thought leader" to their payroll. They have sponsored many of the Phase 3 trials that influence the FDA and the academic environment, even to the extent of influencing the journals and the aggregator establishment that finds gold in the sands of marginal effectiveness. Maybe the stakeholders are not in bed with the FDA and the powers of the academic health center, but they're getting close; they have one foot on the floor.

There is a great deal more to be said about all of this, and I said much of it in my last book, *The Citizen Patient*. Our focus in this book is the environment in which medicine is learned at the level of the trainee or the practicing physician. I teach that whenever one sees a meta-analysis, one should assume that there's much ado about too little to be clinically meaningful—until one is convinced otherwise. However, one hears the conclusions of meta-analyses bandied about in American medicine as if they were pronouncements from Delphi. The more that happens, the more therapeutic decisions degenerate toward the fatuous and the profitable. That means that more often than not, the "translational research" enterprise is sophistry. That means, more often than not, that patients are misinformed and trainees are offered inappropriate role models.

De Morte Medicinae

Transforming "medicine" into the "health-care industry" in the late twentieth century required a major alteration in the infrastructure for the practice of medicine and in the public perception of the need for doing so. Once under way, it did not take long before the transformation invaded the setting for caring, then the examining room itself, and finally the doctor-patient relationship. This chapter and those that follow examine this dialectic stage by stage. However, by taking aim at the doctor-patient relationship, we must not lose sight of the fashion in which the dialectic distances medicine from the needs of the people under the banner "care of the patient" and commandeers the transfer of great wealth in the process. The business of medicine has always influenced the doctor-patient relationship, but now it has come to own it. Furthermore, it is such a big business that it has invoked nearly as much regulatory oversight as the electric power industry. As a result, the doctor-patient relationship is neither privileged nor private; it's as if an auditor and a regulator were participating in every encounter and dominating many.

It is customary to estimate the national investment in health care as a percentage of the Gross Domestic Product (GDP); a number like 17 percent is bandied about, with forecasts approaching 20 percent or more hanging like an imprecation over the economy. These metrics rely heavily on the most accessible costs, usually from the large data banks that collect indemnity costs and other measures of the cash flowing to the purveyors and providers in the health-care industry. But this approach underestimates the money America invests in the quest for "health"; it is more an estimate of the moneys invested in the management of "disease."

Or Is It Health Prevention and Disease Promotion?

Health is much more than the absence of disease. I've devoted several previous books to demonstrating the fine line between the predicaments of life that are personal challenges calling for personal resources for coping and predicaments that are reasonably considered as precursory to, or symptomatic of, disease and therefore worthy of a medical label and medical assistance for coping. This fine line is drawn by consensus; it is a heuristic that reflects common sense and common experience. Contemporary America is focused on and heavily invested in "health" to a degree that spares fewer and fewer of life's predicaments from medicalization. We are willing to run with the scare of the week and the miracle of the month and spend fortunes in the running. For example, a century ago, the common sense held that being overweight, even obese (though not morbidly obese), was a symbol of robust good health. Today, we are to believe that it is anything but. However, contemporary social epidemiology belies both conclusions. It turns out that one's heft, usually expressed as Body Mass Index (BMI), is a surrogate measure of socioeconomic status (SES); the more compromised your SES relative to others in your community, the sooner you are likely to die of something ("all-cause mortality"). That is true today, and it was true in yesteryear. The disaffected, disallowed, and disavowed are at mortal risk regardless of their diet or their girth.

Today, the advantaged live longer, but it has nothing to do with their "healthful lifestyle" or their BMI; it reflects their ability to afford purchases of kale, tofu, Lycra, and the like. The advantaged live longer because they are advantaged. A century ago, a "healthy lifestyle" demanded none of this; to the contrary. The advantaged indulged in many behaviors that today are "health adverse" but were considered health promoting at the time. I'm not saying that either the dietary excesses of the wealthy fin de siècle or the "you can't be too thin" mantra of the wealthy today is preferable; I'm saying that both are irrelevant to their likelihood of dying before their time. Far more relevant is the ability and proclivity to do what one thinks is promoting one's health. Americans are estimated to spend over $32 billion out of pocket each year on vitamins, minerals, botanicals, and all manner of dietary supplements, almost all of which claim benefits that are either unsubstantiated or have proved fatuous. Over 80,000 such products are purveyed in the United States (and elsewhere), requiring no pre-market licensure since the Dietary Supplement Health and Education Act was passed in 1994; if a substance is labeled a dietary supplement, it is to be assumed to be safe until proven otherwise. The FDA is hardly staffed and funded to prove otherwise proactively; hazards are identified after the fact, haphazardly, and sometimes tragically.[1]

I have no doubt that the disparity in people's ability to purchase these putatively salutary products is far more detrimental than the disparity in people's consumption of them. The secret to promoting health in an advantaged society is to allow for access to the mainstream by the less fortunate. This insight is a compelling result of the part of my investigative career that focused on workplace health and safety. It is a major theme in all of my books dating back to the mid-1980s. Today, my work is but one voice in a choir describing, studying, and decrying the adverse consequences of finding oneself in the lower quintiles of socioeconomic status, regardless of how we define socioeconomic status. In a resource-advantaged country, the health consequences of limited opportunity, nonsustaining employment, and social disadvantage are overwhelming. Nonetheless, we remain hell-bent on attacking the surrogates,[2] like BMI and cholesterol, gut/butt ratio, and the lack of physical activities outside of the workplace (regardless of the demands inside). This is another example of missing the forest for the trees, an example that does a great disservice to the informative science, let alone the disadvantaged populace. We know better today,[3] yet we are anchored in the preconceptions of the past.

Health promotion and disease prevention have been quests of all cultures since antiquity, and likewise an ancient venue for scams. However, never before has it co-opted so much of the fabric of daily life and so much of the common sense. Perhaps this speaks to the loosening grip of organized religions, which had long offered up a menu to salve uncertainty that gave medicine's menu a run for its money. Perhaps this speaks to the reach of broadcast and social media. We now have "America's Doctor" and other self-aggrandizing and marketed gurus proclaiming secrets to health to audiences of a size unimaginable to an Elmer Gantry of yore. We have boutique merchants and national grocers hawking all sorts of comestibles as salutary: organic or inorganic, free-range, high in or low in, "green" or native from artichokes and echinacea to zinc. (The last two are representative of the many potions that have no demonstrable benefit when studied systematically.) Then there are all the "wellness" programs that industry underwrites for their workers, a "benefit" many workers would trade for a salary increment if they realized how little these programs advantaged their physical health and how greatly they advantaged the purveyors.[4] Add to this cacophony the proclamations of all the sectarian practitioners who are willing to prod, poke, purge, gird your loins, teach you to breathe or contort, and whatever else for a price and with the conviction that you will be better off for participating. Every conviction is couched in a putative theory communicated with language that sounds sensible and rapidly becomes familiar. Sectarian beliefs and other alternatives to one's personal resources have long and colorful histories, but never before were they so intrusive and pervasive.

Several years ago, I published my first "Four Laws of Therapeutic Dynamics"; the third law is: "There has never been a quack without a theory."[5] I'd venture to say that American "health" expenditures in the first decade of the twenty-first century have captured far more than the usual estimate of 17 percent of the GDP, perhaps twice that if we define health this broadly. Furthermore, the percentage of the population that purchases or purveys health, or does both, has grown to be enormous during the course of the decade, approaching the ubiquitous. We have become a worried society prone to medicalization and willing to expend time and money for any of the many putative solutions that might strike our fancy. We won't leap to purchasing the Brooklyn Bridge or buy faulty manufactured products more than once, but when it comes to health, we are patsies. We are particularly willing if others are sharing the cost, but we are inclined to budget for them regardless. Our appetite seems boundless for interventions that are not indemnified by health insurance. We have come to believe that more is better. The more the intervention is technologically demanding, expensive, and risky, the more sensible and desirable it seems. And if someone else claims to have been advantaged, particularly if that someone has celebrity, any nagging doubt is banished. All sorts of mainstream, sectarian, alternative, and complementary practitioners populate every fiscally advantaged neighborhood and make inroads into neighborhoods less advantaged. They multiply in their number and in their specialized offering before our eyes. Most appear to be thriving, some impressively, if displays of wealth are truly telling. All of this influences one's perceptions of health and illness. All of this influences one's choice to be a patient and colors one's narrative of illness. Doctors are not immune from hearing all of this, and incorporating some if not most of it into their own perceptions of health. Today, the language of the doctor-patient interaction is replete with sparring idioms, whereas before it was an exercise in linguistic determinism with the doctor in charge.

The Sick Citadels

In 1946, shortly after ascending to the presidency, Harry Truman signed the Hospital Survey and Construction Act—the Hill-Burton Act—into law. The Hill-Burton Act underwrote a state-based initiative to build as many hospitals as it took to provide 4.5 beds per 1,000 people. Rural America was soon dotted with small medical centers. As the millennium approached, these started to disappear, a trend that continues to this day. They are supplanted by sizable regional medical centers, some new but many great expansions of medical centers that had long served urban America. Wherever they are located, this new generation of medical centers has come to be a major, if not the primary, source of employment in their regions. This reflects both the decline in labor-intensive traditional industries and the extraordinary growth of the health industry. It is estimated that about one in eight Americans are employed in the health-care industry, some 16 million jobs supporting over 50 million people. The only sector of the economy that is more labor intense is retail trades. Furthermore, the U.S. Department of Commerce predicts that jobs in home health-care services and diagnostic laboratories will grow by nearly 40 percent over the next decade. If the trend continues, a majority of Americans will be providers and/or recipients of health care at any given time.

Most of the American medical centers are no longer hospitals; they are networks of inpatient and outpatient facilities that compete with one another, market aggressively, display grandiose titles, and vie for the most recognizable logo. These systems represent the second attempt to adhere to the mantra perpetrated by yet another burgeoning New Age component of the "health" industry: health-care management consulting firms. The common wisdom of these consultants is a variation of the principle of economy of scale; a hospital system must

De Morte Medicinae

commandeer the care of a very large number of patients so that the few among them who require highly specialized care can be funneled to the providers in the system. Much of these prized patients require diagnostic and surgical procedures that can be centralized in the system. These specialized diagnostic and surgical procedures generate the substantial cash flow necessary to support the enterprise. Structuring the system in this fashion is a form of systems engineering that serves more than economies of scale; it promotes herding of the cash cows.

In the first iteration of this business model in the 1990s, major hospitals started to buy up primary-care private practices, independent clinics, and specialized treatment facilities. The consultants applauded. Various accountants and other number crunchers would look at the patient mix and cash flow of the practices they were acquiring and readily justify a hefty purchase price. As an unanticipated consequence, many a purchasing institution was nearly or actually bankrupted by these acquisitions. Many were forced to sell their entire facility or part of their facility to private-sector corporations that seemed to have mastered the business of consolidation. Some prominent and major institutions met this fate; the teaching hospitals of Georgetown University and the University of Louisville are examples. The University of Pennsylvania Hospital System found itself in dire financial straits after its chief executive officer, William Kelley, M.D., pursued this course. (Bill Kelley had a distinguished career in academic medicine before he chose to transition to mogul.)

The usual reason offered by the world of health economics and by "Wall Street" for the failure of the model is that in relinquishing ownership, the physicians had less incentive to perform at the same pace. In other words American physicians are largely driven by income and by pride of ownership. If that's true, it must pertain only to American physicians, since European physicians manage to achieve better "care" in terms of societal health despite working largely in state-owned facilities and on salary. Are American physicians so libertarian that they can't work for the "man"? Or is a business model that elevates economy of scale fatally flawed? Could it be that it deprived American physicians of the rewards inherent in relationships with their patients? Or could it be that the administrative costs of operating these corporate entities, including profitability, exceeded the savings from sharing the expenses of the practices themselves? Many of these corporate entities were for-profit companies, some even publicly traded. Even the "not-for-profit" designation does not preclude a drive for bloated administrative earnings. The consultants and the administrators were not leaping to accept any of the blame.

The second iteration is ongoing. The hospital consulting firms, whose employees are often enticed with generous salaries to remain on the administrative staff of their clients, adjusted their advising. The best way to avoid the consequences of disincentives is for health-care systems to build new facilities or purchase older facilities and staff them with their own employees. It is an approach that has sounded the death knell for the community hospitals that were the legacy of the Hill-Burton Act. It is also the approach that explains the proliferation of outpatient clinics and the expansion of the mother hospitals. Today, the "all-American crossroads" has a clinic on one corner, a fast-food restaurant on another, and competing drug stores on the remaining two. And today, the all-American hospital system is highly leveraged and dependent on escalating fees for its services if its administration is to enjoy the largesse to which it has grown accustomed.

McKinsey and Company is a ninety-year-old, New York–based global management consulting behemoth. Two of its most senior executives were convicted of federal charges of insider trading in 2012. The brand seems to have recovered. McKinsey remains a very influential advisor to senior executives in nearly all of the major corporations across many industries, including health care. McKinsey has developed the McKinsey Global Institute (MGI), a collaboration with academicians, mainly economists, that collects and analyzes data and produces reports designed to inform corporate decision making. Many wander onto the Internet and into the public sector, where they fuel management wisdom and stimulate consultations by McKinsey analysts. The health-care industry is a major client, and many MGI reports find their way into PowerPoint presentations in the administrative conference rooms of the stakeholders in the health-care industry. For example, a 2011 report titled "Big Data: The Next Frontier for Innovation, Competition, and Productivity"[6] takes the notion of the "Electronic Medical Record" to heights we will discuss shortly.

"Accounting for the Cost of U.S. Health Care: A New Look at Why Americans Spend More" was released in 2008 based on 2006 data.[7] PowerPoint slides from the report have been downloaded and pepper more than boardroom presentations; they can be found in all sorts of media presentations and in commentaries in the medical literature. Many of the report's conclusions have become common wisdom in administrative circles. For example, it found outpatient care to be much more cost-efficient than inpatient care, justifying the explosion in off-site, procedure-oriented clinics. It also found administrative costs to be better than expected given the need for the American health-care system to march to many different legislated and regulatory drums. The report's authors considered U.S. administrative costs, some of which are five times the amount spent by our nearest competitors, a surprising bargain. They apparently had expected the U.S. costs to be $19 billion more than they calculated. One implication is that U.S. health care might be better served if even more was expended on administration, and management consultations might be advisable as to the spending.

I am no stranger to econometrics, having spent much time with the literature on labor economics as a student of workplace health and safety. Econometrics is at a disadvantage because it depends almost exclusively on administrative data sets. At least for some questions in biostatistics, we can try to validate the administrative data by sampling the population directly. We often learn that the administrative data was insufficiently comprehensive or fine structured to offer the insights we seek with any reliability, let alone validity. For example, it is known that the majority of registered nurses employed in American health centers do not directly care for patients; they have all sorts of administrative, educational, and quality-control roles. Do we know whether the econometricians who are defining administrative costs consider "nurses" as administrators or as providers of health services? This question pertains to many categories of employee in the American medical industry.

Hospital Administration as Systems Engineering Gone Mad

Once this process commenced, it took no time at all, less than a decade, for the country to stand agape as its "hospitals" were transformed into behemoths, each hell-bent to increase their "market share" as if they were designed to sell health rather than provide health care. Today, the "hospital" is often a conglomeration of multiple inpatient facilities

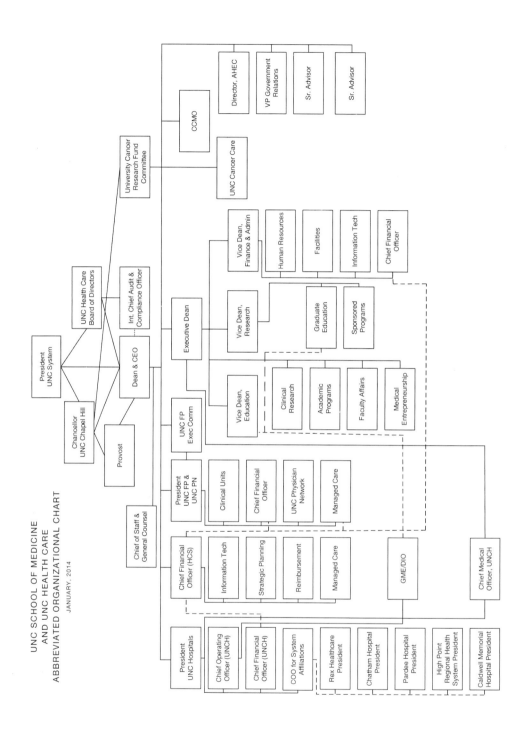

UNC SCHOOL OF MEDICINE
AND UNC HEALTH CARE
ABBREVIATED ORGANIZATIONAL CHART

JANUARY, 2014

President UNC System

Chancellor UNC Chapel Hill

UNC Health Care Board of Directors

Provost

Dean & CEO

Int. Chief Audit & Compliance Officer

Executive Dean

University Cancer Research Fund Committee

CCMO

UNC Cancer Care

Director, AHEC

VP Government Relations

Sr. Advisor

Sr. Advisor

Vice Dean, Finance & Admin

Human Resources

Facilities

Information Tech

Chief Financial Officer

Vice Dean, Research

Graduate Education

Sponsored Programs

Vice Dean, Education

Clinical Research

Academic Programs

Faculty Affairs

Medical Entrepreneurship

UNC FP Exec Comm

President UNC FP & UNC PN

Clinical Units

Chief Financial Officer

UNC Physician Network

Managed Care

Chief of Staff & General Counsel

Chief Financial Officer (HCS)

Information Tech

Strategic Planning

Reimbursement

Managed Care

GME/DIO

Chief Medical Officer, UNCH

President UNC Hospitals

Chief Operating Officer (UNCH)

Chief Financial Officer (UNCH)

COO for System Affiliations

Rex Healthcare President

Chatham Hospital President

Pardee Hospital President

High Point Regional Health System President

Caldwell Memorial Hospital President

De Morte Medicinae

differentiated by clinical purview ("Children's Hospital," "Cancer Hospital," etc.), spawning multiple off-site clinics serving particular clinical specializations. Buildings sprout devoted to the centralization of procedures: imaging centers, gastroscopy centers, outpatient surgery centers, clinical laboratories, and on and on. Other buildings house support for the burgeoning administrations of the various components, central administrative buildings that often are placed at some distance from anything directly related to patient care.

The American "health-care system" is a conglomeration of multiples of these complex "hospitals," each serving a different catchment area and each surrounded by its supporting casts. Private practitioners are a dying breed, as most capitulate and sign on with the marauding behemoths. The private practitioner has difficulty competing for patients and, more important, generating an income that can support malpractice premiums, facility costs (building and staff), and the expense of complying with the ever-shifting sands of the regulatory climate. Few small practices can meet the demands of all this "overhead" and still generate a comfortable income for the practitioners; better to be a salaried employee and let the "system" deal with the overhead. The exceptions are the private practitioners with lucrative specialties, such as cosmetic dermatologists, ophthalmologists, and endoscopists.

(opposite) FIGURE 2 I was in college when Malvina Reynolds wrote "Little Boxes" and still in college when the late Pete Seeger popularized it. Reynolds wrote it when she saw the sprawling postwar housing developments in Daly City, California, south of San Francisco. The song is a political satire targeting conformity of middle-class America at the time. Today, the same "little boxes" of Daly City are painted a rainbow of vivid colors and occupied largely by an immigrant population from the Philippines. These boxes do not serve conformity as much as they provide a way station for those who are striving to move on to whatever it is they aspire for themselves and their families.

The administrative chart of a typical American health system keeps growing little boxes, each containing a constituency that can be quite sizable. There is mobility within the structure and across to similar structures in other institutions. But this is not a way station; this is an organism with a life of its own and with considerable appetite to grow and acquire. For example, the column of little boxes on the left of the chart has budded more boxes since the summer of 2013. But I already included five boxes, each of which represents an acquired hospital system with its own collection of little boxes. Perhaps a matryoshka doll is a better analogy than a box.

Each component of the health-care system presents administrative challenges, which is served by a purpose-built, on-site bureaucracy. The task of integrating all the local bureaucracies necessitated another bureaucratic tier or two. The organization chart of the modern health center resembles the Pentagon in complexity. The organizational chart for the institution that houses my humble clinical efforts is fairly typical (figure 2). Many of these bureaucrats are titled, often multiply titled, and nearly everyone who is titled has a staff and an office suite. Furthermore, since the administration is self-appointed, self-promoting, and self-aggrandizing, it has little incentive to become "lean and mean." It quickly outgrows available space, funds its own buildings, and distances itself from the actual clinical undertakings of the world it is to oversee. The administration defends its size and turf by proclaiming that it serves as complex an organization as any in government or in the private sector. (Pshaw: the central office of Walmart in Bentonville, Arkansas, is paltry in every dimension when compared with figure 2.) There is always a board of directors, but seldom are the members appointed to see through the fog of putative "health care" in order to recognize what needs to be pared as useless or excessive from the menus of "care" and the bloat of administration. Those who might have this visual acuity have been carefully eliminated in the vetting as unsuitable for the "teamwork" of the sycophancy. This can happen in the private sector, too, but an organization that becomes bloated, lacks direction, is inefficient, and has a flawed output will not survive long in the free market. American health care hides all of this by adopting the shield of "not-for-profit" and proclaiming its value to a market that has no way to validate the claims or favor an alternative. The components of the American health-care system compete in marketing, not in substance. They hawk the "new and better" regardless of efficacy, and they proclaim to be "Number 1" at something even though valid criteria are elusive. When a "system" such as the American health-care "system" loses its way, the result is a perfect storm of ethical bankruptcy. And it has lost its way.

Don't imagine for one moment that the organizing displayed in charts such as figure 2 is following a grand plan, some theoretical model that was generated with efficiency of service and quality of outcome as its goal. Rather, imagine men in green eye shades playing a distorted version of monopoly, acquiring and expanding and building and leveraging. The mother "hospital" for the system depicted in figure 2 (UNCH) has an annual budget of more than $2 billion, about a quarter of which services long-term debt. UNCH is a state-owned entity that managed to accumulate $75 million to purchase Rex Hospital, a 600-plus-bed private not-for-profit hospital in a neighboring city. In fact, the CEO mentioned to the press that UNCH's war chest approached $500 million in case another hospital tried to outbid the offer. UNCH's executive staff is salaried at a level that nearly all other state employees, the governor included, would envy, approaching the incomes of some state "salaried" college football and basketball coaches.

Health-care facilities are scattered helter-skelter across central North Carolina, owned and administered by different "systems" competing for market share. Facilities fly the flags of the Duke HealthCare System out of Durham, the Carolinas Healthcare System out of Charlotte, Cone Health out of Greensboro, and others. Each system employs well over 10,000 workers, about half of whom have access to patient charts. Generally, about 10 to 20 percent of the workforce is comprised of doctoral-level caregivers such as physicians, although the percentage rises to about 30 percent in the academic/research hospitals, where fewer physicians are seeing patients full-time.

This state of affairs is not peculiar to North Carolina. The results of all the buying and building are enormous "systems" all across America. No one is questioning whether all this system building serves anything that anyone might term "health" better than what it is replacing. No doubt it has created all sorts of job categories in response to the unwieldy nature of the organizations and the dispersion of responsibility for the care of the patient. Furthermore, most of these "growth areas" have psychologically, and often physically, distanced themselves so far away from the plight of the patients that those patients are no longer called patients; they are "units of care." And since the cost and debt parameters for the system have grown astronomically, the primary measure of success is in cash flow, which in the current reimbursement system reflects the income per encounter. Hence, "throughput" matters. It is the line of reasoning that succors a fast-food chain. Somebody needs to send another memo to each of the boxes in figure 2, copied to the myriad committees that are attached to each of these boxes, to point out that patients are not hamburgers.

Digital Invoicing

At the beginning of this chapter, I pointed out that the transformation of "medicine" into a "health-care industry" required first creating a different setting for caring. That is fait accompli. Next, it had to intrude into the examining room itself. The coup de grâce is the commandeering of the doctor-patient relationship itself, the topic of the next chapter. The health-care industry took ownership of the examining room by computerizing the clinical interview. This required convincing the country and the federal government that an Electronic Medical Record (EMR) was much more than a confusing, expensive way to garner fees for services. Furthermore, EMR was to be replaced by another acronym, EHR, to denote that matters of "health" were to be recorded, not just "medical" matters.

So, we have administrations in place dedicated to shepherding a wealth of "units of care" to the appropriate front doors in a fashion that optimizes "throughput." That's just for starters. The business model also requires a mechanism to optimize financial return on whatever happens to each unit on the way through. That requires efficient invoicing. The units of care and/or their underwriters must be billed for all services and moneys collected in as expeditious a fashion as possible. No longer does this mean "as humanly possible."

Over the course of the five decades we are considering in this book, reimbursement for medical and surgical treatment has undergone a sea change. It started with a fee-for-service that countenanced a scale from charity care to "soak the rich." This approach came to a screeching halt with the introduction of Medicare and the growth of private health insurance. But the screeching halt was possible only after a compromise between the Johnson administration and organized medicine, which was then represented largely by the American Medical Association (AMA). The compromise was that in return for supporting this incursion of "socialized medicine," the AMA would be charged with defining the evaluations and management interventions that were to be covered. Furthermore, the AMA was charged with the establishment of a fee scale so that reimbursement would remain "usual and customary." A good deal of my last book, *Citizen Patient*, is a detailed discussion of this contract and the unintended consequences that became apparent after a lag of nearly a decade. Here, a brief overview will suffice to bring us to the conundrum of the unintended consequences for patient care of the contemporary solutions.

To serve the compromise, the AMA was charged with creating a listing of procedures that Medicare should underwrite. An Editorial Panel was chosen from the membership and the compendium of Current Procedural Terminology (CPT) was first published in 1966. The panel has met three times a year ever since to consider changes in "Evaluation/Management Services" (E/M); an updated compendium is released each October. Recent editions contain more than 10,000 E/M codes. No longer is a doctor to simply see a patient or lance a boil; there are separate codes for the elements of evaluations, procedures, and other aspects of management. Furthermore, reimbursement is negotiated with Medicare and private insurance companies on a piecemeal basis. The coding can be complex, and reimbursement is highly dependent on the degree to which the coding manages to capture every possible charge. As a result, "coding" has become an allied health profession and a major curriculum in community colleges. Any sizable hospital employs hundreds of coders. They also employ individuals who "audit" the coding, as do the various payers—despite which, notorious examples of fraud have come to light.

It did not take long for the Medicare administration to realize that paying hospitals fee-for-service on a piecemeal basis was inefficient. It made more sense to pay for a "product," a conglomeration of services for a clinical entity. One might pay for an appendectomy rather than each element of the evaluation and management of appendicitis. The result was the development of another compendium of "Disease-Related Groups" (DRGs). The first one had 467 DRGs. It was tested in a couple of states and launched nationally in the mid-1980s. DRG #467 was for an "ungroupable" category. The original assumption was that there were 466 clinical events that are so homogeneous and predictable that a prospective payment system could replace cost-based hospital reimbursement. The hospital is paid based on the DRG; if the patient sails through the procedure, the profit margin increases and vice versa. Of course, a patient might qualify for more than one DRG or for a more complex DRG if the illness is confounded or treatment leads to complications. Furthermore, the number of DRGs has expanded greatly over time, but not enough to eliminate an "ungroupable" category.

DRGs take advantage of the International Statistical Classification of Diseases and Related Health Problems (ICD) established by the World Health Organization long ago and upgraded periodically. DRGs are currently based on the ICD-9 listing of some 17,000 clinical conditions. Coding starts with a particular ICD-9 label (sometimes more than one) that is captured by a particular DRG upon which reimbursement is based. In March 2014 the United States was to have adopted the ICD-10 for this purpose, but the wonks thought better of that start-up date given the chaos of implementing other aspects of the Affordable Care Act. The start-up was postponed.

The ICD-9 is a compendium of diagnostic labels. The ICD-10 has over 155,000 categories of disease and is built on a different principle, which is illustrated in the example that follows. The first letter is the general category; the "W" indicates any external cause of the symptoms that is not captured by another category, and the "S" indicates that the external cause was an injury. The numbers and letters of each code are a chain of descriptions that hones down to the particulars of causes and effects.

THE CODER'S DILEMMA

A young woman has slipped and fallen on ice, injuring her tailbone (coccyx). There is no exact ICD-10 code. The coder must pick from:

W00 Fall due to ice and snow
W00.0 Fall on same level due to ice and snow
W00.0xxA Fall on same level due to ice and snow, initial
    encounter
W00.0xxD Fall on same level due to ice and snow, subsequent
    encounter
W00.0xxS Fall on same level due to ice and snow, sequela
W00.1 Fall from stairs and steps due to ice and snow
W00.1xxA Fall from stairs and steps due to ice and snow, initial
    encounter

W00.1xxD Fall from stairs and steps due to ice and snow, subsequent encounter

W00.1xxS Fall from stairs and steps due to ice and snow, sequela

W00.2 Other fall from one level to another due to ice and snow

W00.2xxA Other fall from one level to another due to ice and snow, initial encounter

W00.2xxD Other fall from one level to another due to ice and snow, subsequent encounter

W00.2xxS Other fall from one level to another due to ice and snow, sequela

W00.9 Unspecified fall due to ice and snow

W00.9xxA Unspecified fall due to ice and snow, initial encounter

W00.9xxD Unspecified fall due to ice and snow, subsequent encounter

W00.9xxS Unspecified fall due to ice and snow, sequela

There are also codes for ice skating and hockey injuries. If the coccyx is fractured, S32.2 so indicates; additional numbers/letters expand the diagnosis to indicate aspects of the clinical course:

S32.2 Fracture of coccyx

S32.2xxA Fracture of coccyx, initial encounter for closed fracture

S32.2xxB Fracture of coccyx, initial encounter for open fracture

S32.2xxD Fracture of coccyx, subsequent encounter for fracture with routine healing

S32.2xxG Fracture of coccyx, subsequent encounter for fracture with delayed healing

S32.2xxK Fracture of coccyx, subsequent encounter for fracture with nonunion

That's a lot of "granularity" for just slipping on your butt.

The argument for the ICD-10 is that it creates an even-more-detailed basis for billing and an enormous data set that is sufficiently detailed, "granular," to support studies of the effectiveness of interventions in practice, so-called comparative effectiveness research. The introduction of the Electronic Health Record utilizing ICD-9 categorization has proved both expensive and chaotic. It is reassuring to learn that the powers that be, in a fleetingly lucid moment, thought better of superimposing ICD-10 on the challenges of introducing the Electronic Health Record across the country. Shortly, we will be discussing whether either promise of granularity is more than fatuous.

CPTs and DRGs are the attempt to constrain the "open season" for billing for the activities that go into the stuff of evaluation and management. Medicare administration soon realized it had the same challenge in serving the mandate to pay physicians their "usual and customary" fees for evaluating and managing patients. William Hsiao, a professor of economics at the Harvard School of Public Health, was recruited to the task. He obliged by creating the Resource-Based Relative Value Scale (RBRVS), which was codified in the Omnibus Budget Reconciliation Act signed into law by President George H. W. Bush in 1988. For every CPT, a fee was to be determined based principally on physicians' experience and cost of practice prorated, recently, for the cost of malpractice insurance. In the early 1990s, with some input from various lobbyists, Medicare administration turned to its old friend, the AMA, for guidance regarding implementation. In 1991 the AMA established the Specialty Society RBRVS Update Committee (RUC) for this task. The RUC has twenty-nine members, twenty-three appointed by specialty professional societies and three by the AMA itself. The committee is heavily weighted to surgeons and other interventionalists who unabashedly consider their activities high on the RBRVS. I am no longer alone in demanding a reexamination of the notion of "value" in this context.[8] Currently, "value" remains in the eyes of the beholders on the RUC; it needs to be reframed as in the eyes of the recipient. I don't care how valuable the doctors think they are; their compensation should reflect the value they add to the quality and duration of the life of the patient. As I have written on many other occasions, so much that extravagantly advantages providers often disadvantages patients to a comparable degree.

Economists reserve the term "regulatory capture" to describe the circumstance where a public regulatory agency is controlled by the interests it is meant to regulate. But that's too highfalutin a term. How about "corrupt" and "immoral"? The driver for maintaining the current approach is its profitability for myriad stakeholders, including the private insurance industry, who drive stakes with relentless lobbying and by liberally applying largesse to buy support and maintain conflictual relationships. "Gaming" the system has become a national pastime. The push-back from the federal government comes mainly from tweaking the regulations governing Medicare reimbursements under the banner of quality of care. If patients return to the hospital soon after discharge for the same DRG, there is a penalty. If the hospitalization is prolonged because of iatrogenicity, complications of care that should have been avoided, there is a penalty. You can imagine how the energies of coders and auditors are co-opted by these incompatible agendas; the "providers" wish to maximize income runs into Medicare's feeble attempt to control cost. The gaming can be demonstrated easily; secondary gain influences the way patients admitted to hospital with pneumonia are coded.[9]

Rather than argue for a complete revamping, for a novel approach that takes advantage of any of the single-payer, national health insurance schemes employed abroad, America is seeking a solution in analytics. The Affordable Care Act does not assault the Babel of invoicing. To the contrary. The solution currently being offered is buried in the Electronic Health Record, which is already mandatory for larger institutions and will be universal before long if the federal government has its way. These are computer programs that require providers to enter actions and codes leading to large data sets with the "granularity" that is considered the secret to efficient invoicing. The ICD-10 appeals to this mindset, but even with the ICD-9, a patient encounter or admission can send myriad data points into the maw of invoicing. I'm not surprised that it has proved difficult to demonstrate that the implementation of the EHR leads to a reduction in costs[10] or any other impressive utility,[11] even in outpatient settings.[12] But the EHR has its stakeholders; some are wonks with their policy prowess at risk, and others are stockholders with deep pockets. All are crying "wait and see," even the current crop of RAND Corporation thought leaders.[13]

RAND is an acronym for Research ANd Development. The corporation was established after World War II by the Douglas Aircraft Company as a nonprofit think tank dedicated to serving policy and strategy needs relating to national defense and welfare. The latter expanded to a major investment in policy and strategy relating to the health of the population. Much of this effort is driven by economic and systems considerations distant from the bedside, though RAND is not averse to conducting or sponsoring relevant research. The influence of RAND on health policy is impressive and, in retrospect, impressively inconsistent in terms of farsightedness and beneficence. It was a RAND study that purported to demonstrate how "co-pay" decreases utilization and thereby costliness without an analysis of the downstream risks for individual patients. And it is RAND that called for the widespread adoption of health information technology in 2005 promising great improvements in efficiency and safety. A cost savings was estimated at more than $80 billion annually based on sophisticated econometric modeling.[14] So much for soothsaying based on unproved assumptions. The effect on cost has been paradoxical. The effect on quality of care has been inconsistent[15] but never compellingly demonstrated, according to RAND investigators.[16] Even for something as seemingly straightforward as medications, "computerized provider order entry" (CPOE) does not appear to reduce prescribing errors.[17]

Nonetheless, "granularity" remains the rallying cry. Big data should render the invoicing predictable and reliable, though not necessarily valid. What matters is that all charges capture what was actually done, not whether there is price gouging—let alone whether the cost provided value in terms of benefit to the patient. No one is exercised over the fact that any test, drug, procedure, visit, or whatever can cost many times more in one setting than in another. No one is exercised over the fact that the charges for any of these can be many times greater than the actual costs. What matters most to Medicare is that no bill is submitted for services that were never rendered, and what matters most to the providers is that no service goes unbilled. The notion of "usual and customary" fees operates beyond physician fees; it institutionalizes a costing of CPTs as varied and opaque as the bad old days of whatever-the-trade-will-bear, fee-for-service medicine. The striking variability in invoicing across geographic regions for Medicare pales next to the variability in the private sector, even for consumable supplies, from bandages to food supplies. The variability in provider charges to Medicare is even more striking than the geographic variations. In 2012 nearly 900,000 individual providers billed Medicare for some $2.5 billion; only a third of that sum was qualified for payment, averaging $87,000 per provider. However, some 2,000 providers broke

$2 million; the top ten received a combined $121 million for Medicare Part B payments.[18]

But the EHR is a feature of every patient encounter in every medical center and in an ever-growing number of smaller practices. Big Brother is there. And it is such a presence that the conversation between a doctor and a patient is no longer a dialogue.

Missing the Forest for
the Granularity

"Going to the doctor" today is not your grandfather's experience. In all likelihood, you'll park in a deck, walk through a marble lobby, and report to a secretary behind a counter who is pretending to make your approach anonymous. Then you'll take a seat and wait to be called for "intake": questionnaire, vital signs, review of medications—and the back of the head of the intaker, usually a nurse, as he hovers over the computer. You may wait in the lobby further until called into your doctor's examining room. The greeting is warm, cordial, and brief before she turns away to also hover over the computer. Care of the patient in the current system demands attention to the requirements of the Electronic Health Record; much must be entered and given time constraints, much needs to be entered in real time. This is so intrusive that many institutions are providing their providers with assistance in the form of "scribes" who do the entering into the appropriate places demanded by the program as the information is elicited. That preserves a vestige of eye contact. It might seem that you and your doctor are in the room to serve the entry of data. It might seem so because it is nearly so.

The rationale behind the EHR seems obvious. Medicine has been generating escalating reams of paper documentation for decades. Clinical records, billing records, and all sorts of process records created endless paper trails. Retrieving information was as difficult as storing it. And transferring information across boundaries was time-consuming and costly. Furthermore, this was anything but a reliable form of record keeping. Illegible and incorrect notes and entries were difficult to identify in real time, let alone in retrospect. Starting late in the twentieth century, this situation challenged information technology to produce a solution; many resulted. The paper record was largely replaced by digital records that attempted to reproduce the form and intent of the traditional record. Human errors were not totally eliminated; the data was only as reliable as the entry event. But the mountains of paper disappeared, and the challenges for retrieval were greatly improved. Transferability remained a problem given the multiplicity of computer programs. But that was not the driver to the next generation of EHRs.

The driver was the argument that digitized medical information is a rich source of information that could be mined for many purposes if it was in an accessible format. In particular, it could be mined to fine-tune invoicing and to examine the utilities of elements of patient care. As part of the 2009 American Recovery and Reinvestment Act (the economic "stimulus" act), the Obama administration invested a great deal of money in response to this argument. We will consider the impact this agenda is having on the doctor-patient relationship shortly. First, let's examine the agenda that calls for aggregating data from multiple patients to compare the effectiveness of various interventions.

Comparative Effectiveness Research and Kindred Delusions

Granularity and "big data" are held up as the solution for the mystery of effectiveness. It is hoped that by analyzing large data sets, one could identify approaches to evaluation and to management (E/M) that have too little utility in practice in the population at large to justify their application and/or cost. This is meant to supplement the mission of the FDA. The FDA has stringent requirements for the licensure of drugs, but less-stringent ones for the licensure of devices and none for procedures. The licensure of drugs is dependent on a demonstration of *efficacy*, not *effectiveness*. The prerequisite of efficacy is met when a new drug is associated with more benefit than a placebo in a randomized controlled trial lasting months, occasionally longer, and generally in highly defined populations of volunteers. The result is a statistical construct; the benefit is observed more frequently than one would predict by chance alone. It does not stipulate anything more— nothing about the magnitude or duration of the benefit, the actual frequency the benefit is to be expected, or whether the result generalizes to individuals who do not meet the requirements for volunteering. Randomized controlled trials are expensive, difficult undertakings that are more likely to be informative as the population studied becomes less heterogeneous. We might learn whether the new drug advantages men or women, the young or old, patients with only one disease or with many, and the like. Licensure often reflects these limitations of the licensing trials, but postlicensure marketing often tests these limits, and prescription is not at all regulated accordingly. Postlicensure drugs join devices and procedures in the general therapeutic milieu with the proclamation that one size fits all, but no assurance that one size fits any but the particular population studied in the licensing randomized controlled trial.

"Granularity" comes to the rescue? Is there a way to look at the experience in practice and deduce some more general notion of effectiveness? In epidemiology speak, "efficacy" pertains to the results of a systematic study on a highly selected target population, a randomized controlled trial; "effectiveness" pertains to outcomes in more usual practice. Building on work initiated in the "stimulus" act, the Patient Protection and Affordable Care Act created the Patient-Centered Outcomes Research Institute (PCORI) to "answer real-world questions about what works best for patients based on their particular circumstances and concerns. We do this primarily by funding comparative clinical effectiveness research (CER) studies that compare multiple care options."[1] Joe Selby, M.D., M.P.H., is a family physician and an accomplished epidemiologist who spent many years in both roles at Kaiser Permanente before being recruited as the executive director of PCORI. I have long had, and published,[2] reservations about the potential of CER to parse meaningful insights from data that is heterogeneous in accuracy, validity, and quality, regardless of how "big" the data are. Perhaps a recent exchange between Joe Selby and me will serve to give the reader the gist of the argument. This exchange occurred in response to an essay posted on The Health Care Blog (THCB), perhaps the most read and most influential of the blogs that captures the attention of those with a particular interest in health-policy matters. The posting and all comments are archived (http://thehealthcareblog.com/blog/2014/03/27/how-pcoris-research-will-answer-the-questions-patients-are-asking/).

1. NORTIN HADLER TO JOE SELBY: I applaud the premise behind CER and therefore the rationale for PCORI. However, I have grave concerns that the effort is largely doomed by methodological challenges. I expressed these reservations on THCB shortly after the creation of PCORI and nothing has assuaged my concerns to date: http://www.thehealthcareblog.com/the_health_care_blog/2010/01/comparative-effectiveness-research-and-kindred-delusions.html#more.

In essence, I don't think any degree of data torturing can compensate for the marginal efficacy of so many targets for CER. If the efficacy in a carefully selected subset of patients is marginal (NNT >50 or 100 or . . .), you run the risk of comparative ineffectiveness research. CER only makes sense if it can be anchored in a relevant example of efficacy in some subset.

Examples of marginal efficacy are legion, such as oral hypoglycemics, statins, many cancer screening protocols, and much more, including highly marketed fads such as the stenting of STEMIs (http://thehealthcareblog.com/blog/2013/10/13/the-end-of-the-coronary-angioplasty-era/) and anti-coagulants for nonvalvular A-fib (http://thehealthcareblog.com/blog/2014/02/01/why-your-a-fib-diagnosis-may-not-be-as-bad-as-you-think-it-is/).

Of course, this concern would not pertain to comparative *cost* research, but that is explicitly disallowed in the legislation and therefore is not a PCORI agenda.

2. JOE SELBY TO NORTIN HADLER: I agree. Comparative effectiveness studies are often done in situations where expected differences are small or where the expectation is that there is no difference—difficult territory to operate in, but nonetheless important. We also agree that comparative effectiveness research is complementary to and usually follows on the establishment of efficacy and even effectiveness. Three points may offer some comfort. First, a major problem when differences are small is that it's hard to discern true differences from apparent differences that are due to selection bias (confounding), especially in non-randomized studies. That's why nearly half of all PCORI studies and nearly all of the larger studies we're funding are randomized trials. Second, although differences for some outcomes may be

small or nonexistent, they may be larger for others, like side effects or quality of life. That's why PCORI emphasizes considering a broader range of outcomes than in typical efficacy studies. And third, "marginal" effects often result from studying heterogeneous populations that contain subgroups who benefit differentially and subgroups who don't—so the average effect is "marginal." PCORI emphasizes and expects funded research to pay special attention to possible differences in relative effectiveness within a study population, and to seek to identify those patients who benefit a lot from making a particular choice and those in whom the choice doesn't matter or is reversed. This is the patient-centered approach: learning what works better for whom, for the outcomes that matter most to them.

I suspect that PCORI will spend down its budget and produce a good deal of data that, on analysis, offers little that should be considered compelling to a patient and a doctor coming together to try to make a particular decision. It is very difficult to control for the variability in individuals in a large data set when the variables are defined and measured; there is no way to take into account the variables that were not or could not be measured.

Dr. Big Brother

EPIC is a privately held software company founded by Judith Faulkner in 1979 and headquartered near Madison, Wisconsin. As a graduate student at the University of Wisconsin in Madison, Faulkner took advantage of an older platform, MUMPS, the "Multi-User Multi-Programming System" developed at the Massachusetts General Hospital, to write the software that was to evolve into EPIC. EPIC engineers subsequently developed a suite of health-care software designed to service the needs of large health-care organizations. Without the benefit of outside capital or even marketing, "Judy" Faulkner grew her company into a behemoth and her personal wealth into the billions of dollars. EPIC and several other companies, such as Cerner, were poised to take advantage of the Health Information Technology for Economic and Clinical Health (HI TECH) agenda that was a $19 billion pot tucked into the 2009 stimulus bill designed to create new jobs. HI TECH legislation forced the development of health information technology with both carrots and sticks: the introduction of electronic medical records was directly subsidized and further promoted by the threat of a cut in Medicare reimbursement to any hospital that could not demonstrate its "meaningful use" of the Electronic Health Record by 2015. EPIC landed the Kaiser Health System as a client and has come to dominate the large-institution market, implementing its software suite at a cost of hundreds of millions per institution. The landing of the Kaiser System, for $4 billion, a decade ago is the stuff of legend.[3] Cleveland Clinic, Johns Hopkins, most institutions in the University of California system, and others have made EPIC the dominant provider of electronic medical records in the country.

My institution, UNC Health Care, undertook transition to the EPIC system in 2014. I held off writing this chapter until UNCH "went live" in the spring and I'd stopped reeling from the experience. Every "provider" was required to take >20 hours of classroom instruction and many more hours of online instruction. Many took additional instruction to become "super-users" who would provide hand-holding when we "went live." The faculty and staff were expected to travel off-site to a converted shopping mall for all the mandatory classes. All our hardware was replaced with the EPIC-compatible hardware. Over 1,000 EPIC "qualified" instructors took up residence in Chapel Hill and circulated in our clinical arena, holding the hands that "super-users" did not or could not accommodate. Patient care and all else of that sort was subjugated to the implementation of EPIC. It was/is truly an awesome exercise in theater of the absurd. It is also unconscionably costly. This is an exercise that tossed the hospitals affiliated with Wake Forest University Medical School so deep into debt that many employees had to be laid off. It is an exercise that has caused UNCH to trim all sorts of budgets and initiate contingency layoff plans. It is the straw that may break the back of America's perverse health-care system.

It is also an outrageously misguided exercise. No doubt the promise of billing efficiency co-opted reasoning and suppressed forewarnings from clinical staff. However, clinical staff around the country now speak, sotto voce, to an administration that is in control. The "suits" that contracted EPIC were of like mind across much of the hospital firmament. This clumsy approach to invoicing trades off the essence of clinical medicine: the elicitation of the patient's narrative, its parsing, and the recording of both for the sake of continuity of care. EPIC demands that sufficient information is entered to satisfy the demands of coding, auditing, and "meaningful usage." The latter demands that superficial clinical details, most of which are obvious to the patient, be recorded and a document, the After Visit Summary (AVS), produced and handed to the patient before leaving the office. Entering the data required for coding and for the AVS is a complex task that is anything but intuitive. It requires familiarity with a very detailed and redundant computer interface, and even then it is time-consuming. I schedule follow-up visits in twenty-minute slots, which I devote, almost entirely, to face-to-face encounters with my patients. When, or if, I tame EPIC, I will still have to devote much of the time slot to face-to-interface medicine, or add that task to the work of an already tightly scheduled week. Practice can make this a more efficient exercise, but there are no shortcuts that spare the cognitive reliability of the clinical record from distortion.

Nonetheless, shortcuts are encouraged in eliciting, recording, and considering the clinical narrative. EPIC encourages, essentially demands, "smart sets." These are templates that assume a degree of stereotyping in clinical encounters, as if some of each patient's experience is common to all patients. So I'm to create, or even borrow from my colleagues, a template that captures the average narrative of a patient with rheumatoid arthritis, or with scleroderma, or with . . . My job is to paste these templates in my patient's record and modify them as I see fit. Worse than that, EPIC encourages cutting and pasting all sorts of prior entries with the click of a button that is meant to assure the material is accurate. This task can be postponed until after the patient leaves the clinic—but not for long after without violating "meaningful usage." However, stereotypes are never referred to me; my patients are individuals. EPIC's algorithms and "smart sets" might be expedient for specialties where the clinical focus is highly discrete conditions, such as for particular procedures. For an orthopedist that operates mainly on shoulders, for example, a template with a blank space for "right or left" might be efficient. My specialty, rheumatology, is considered the proto typical "cognitive" specialty; variations and nuances are the rule. I'll be damned if I will create, borrow, or use "smart sets," and my patients and their referring doctors would be very poorly served if I did.

To add insult to the burden of entering data, EPIC is programmed to "pop up" treatment recommendations. Most are based on guidelines and other consensus statements. The principle is that these statements are so well grounded that they provide the "cookbook" for treatment once the diagnosis is entered. Very few of these consensus statements escape critical review on multiple levels, from the limitations of the clinical science to the biases of the committee that wrote them. Guidelines are at best a guide to clinical debates and to discussions with patients to inform their decisions. Seldom are they the recipe for treatment. All my prior books are replete with examples that support this therapeutic posture. For many of the diagnoses that I frequently make, the recommendations and discussions that pop up are highly debatable and can be inappropriate prescriptions. The advice for backache and its variants are a particularly egregious example I am often forced to ignore.

Treating through EPIC means that "cognitive" physicians devote an inordinate amount of time and energy to their computers. It is so burdensome and tiresome that many physicians, even those in procedure-based specialties, are demanding the creation of yet another allied health profession: the "scribes." These are people who are trained to sit by the side of the physician as the clinical narrative unfolds and perform computer entry. Scribes make it feasible for cognitive clinicians to engage in the intimate, trusting encounter that makes clinical care possible. Scribes are now handmaidens to the physicians staffing our Emergency Department at UNC; without them, our Emergency Department physicians could not attend to our relatively gentle rush of patients. Without scribes, even the most cognitive of cognitive physicians have learned to suppress their cognition long enough to treat their computers. If one rounds in the American hospital today, it is easy to find doctors at the computer, but they are as rare as hens' teeth at the bedside. The notion is that others can record at the bedside; the physician is Oz the "Wizard"—not "America's doctor" Oz, the Wizard wannabe, but the allegorical wizard—sequestered, collecting data, and organizing the fate of others.

For forty years, I kept my own patient charts under lock and key and with the begrudging sanction of UNCH. During the course of a patient encounter, I would create a handwritten record of my clinical observations with a writing paper that automatically made a copy.

The original went into the paper record of old, the copy into a green folder that was filed in my office. Before we had computerized records, the original scribblings were the hospital record accompanied by the long letter I would dictate to the referring doctor and copied to the patient. Once we had the first generation of computerized records, I modified the dictation, but only slightly, so that the letter became the sole record of the encounter. These were designed to be comprehensive and instructional. They were available to anyone else—an emergency-room doctor, for example, with a need to understand my thinking about the patient. But the green folders remained an important ancillary source for me in caring for the patient over time. These are where I also recorded information about the patient's life events that were not directly related to his primary disease, information such as the name of his newborn daughter, his spouse's challenges, and the like. I also stored the notes and missives from his doctors so that they would be available at the time of a follow-up; seldom could the hospital record department scan these materials into the digital record in a sufficiently timely manner. These "shadow charts" supplemented the critical objectivity of the hospital charts with the tidbits that spoke to the idiosyncrasies of my patient's life. I carried these folders to clinic.

Composing the letter to the referring and other treating doctors, which was always copied to the patient, was as important a part of the encounter as any other. The letter served the need to document the clinical course, the life context in which it played out, my thinking about diagnosis and management, and the literature that I found informative. These letters were as comprehensive as the encounter demanded. If anyone needed to know the patient's clinical status and my thinking at the time of the encounter, these letters were forever a ready resource; they became my entry into the chart. I continued this practice after UNCH did away with personal secretaries, meaning that I spent more and more time editing the work product of various transcriptionists or even computerized transcription. I felt this was an obligation, not a task, and I took great pride in my prose.

The letters may have done justice to patient care, but they slowly came to serve invoicing less and less expediently. However, accurate invoicing is far from my top priority; I was called on the carpet more than once for "underbilling." With the advent of EPIC, the green folders and these letters were rendered obsolete, sacrificed to the granularity of the Electronic Health Record and its compliance with administrative mandates. I was determined to try to serve my patients as long as I could serve them according to my conscience. That goal and my sense of humor were being tested, sorely.

Subliminal Marketing

The required online training for EPIC included a gratuitous course designed to make all clinical personal aware of a clinical condition that required immediate attention. There is a form of heart attack—a STEMI—notable for a particular finding on an electrocardiogram. We are to assume that anyone who looks particularly ill, even in the lobby of the hospital, with or without chest pain, has a STEMI until proved otherwise with an electrocardiogram. We are to alert the "STEMI Team" to make the determination and, if a STEMI is diagnosed, to whisk the patient off for cardiac catheterization and, if feasible, the placement of a stent in the offending coronary artery. Time, we are told, is of the essence if we are to circumvent catastrophe.

This is a perfect example of propaganda masquerading as pedagogy. All stenting is on the thinnest of ice from an evidentiary point of view—including stenting a STEMI.[4] However, propaganda dressed up as authority is no longer just an exercise in "direct-to-consumer" advertising; it is a scourge of the news media and the drumbeat to which health and disease advocacy marches. It is also the soft underbelly of the thousands of guidelines written by "thought leaders" who trip over their conflicts of interest. All this is treated in detail in many of my writings[5] and in the writing of many others, including the Institute of Medicine.[6] Perhaps the most evil example of propaganda masquerading as clinical pedagogy is the insidious introduction of contentious clinical guidance into the Electronic Health Record. Not only are various guidelines and reviews linked to the EHR, but adherence to them also can be monitored digitally—with the assumption that adherence is a measure of "quality of care."

The promulgation of guidelines and other forms of cookbook medicine leads to the conclusion that medicine is a science that is readily reduced to algorithms, roadmaps from diagnosis to cure. There are such algorithms in every Emergency Department, covering myriad acute presentations. There are such in every Intensive Care Unit. In most clinical arenas, the approach has been to provide computerized clinical-decision support systems. The most frequent relate to computerized provider order entry, where various forms of alert pop up when the order violates some sort of standard for dosing or drug-drug interaction. However, for CPOE but also for other aspects of electronic charting, decision monitoring and support programs have proved to have little effectiveness. If there is a role for computers in decision making, it is to facilitate dialogue between patient and physician, not to supplant the input from either[7] or to cut health-care costs.[8]

Sacrificing Care for Efficiency

However, that message is lost in the current digital zeal. Rather, time at the bedside, patient-doctor dialogue, breadth of experience, range of interests, or time to consider and reconsider decisions and uncertainties are increasingly considered charming but antiquated attributes of medicine in the past. Today, efficiency of care is the new frontier, an efficiency that is facilitated by the mechanistic nature of the treatment act. This notion calls into question the essentially humanistic nature of the treatment act. In fact, this notion calls for the elimination of much that I value in the nurturing of physicians who can provide perspective if not wisdom to a fellow human being in need. This notion calls for the targeting of medical education to efficiency. All that I hope might nurture perspective, peer review, critical thinking, and compassion is to be subjugated to getting the tasks done. This encourages a form of cognition that is automatic, reflexive, and intuitive. No doubt this cognitive bias will serve efficiency, but how often will it not serve the patient well, or at all? How often is the presentation atypical, or the narrative skewed by the patient's cognitive bias as to what is "wrong"? How often does uncertainty as to diagnosis and prognosis color the presentation, if not predominate it? The degree to which this is the case is the degree to which the patient is poorly served by mindless medicine.[9]

Nonetheless, reflexive medicine is one of the banners flown by those who advocate for an abbreviation of medical education by truncating medical school to three years.[10] It is argued that no single person can know it all, so why try? Besides, health care is so complex that only well-coordinated teams of individuals, where each member of

Missing the Forest for the Granularity

the team contributes a finely honed and focused skill set, are a match for it.[11] In the next chapter, we will explore why such an intuitive and obvious collaborative model is difficult to implement, if not counterproductive. However, the notion that clustering individuals, each of whom knows more and more about less and less, results in synergy may work in assembly lines and perhaps in the few procedural aspects of medicine that are similarly stereotypical, but it is doomed for most clinical care. There is little about the illness that is predictable in this fashion. Everyone involved in patient care, any aspect of patient care, must be educated to appreciate the limitations of the purview they are to bring to the bedside. Everyone must realize that their particular expertise may not synergize with that of others in the team as much as the limitations of the individual perspectives might synergize. If they don't realize this, we'll have teams of carpenters, each with a hammer in search of what he or she knows to be the nail.

I am arguing that only a clear-thinking and highly educated person can take responsibility for empowering the patient to see through all the uncertainties in order to make informed decisions with self-interest as the goal. I am arguing for a physician to attend truly to that patient, for one who understands the need for a modern version of "The Morning Prayer of the Physician" introduced at the beginning of this book. I am arguing for an education that promulgates this responsible role. However, my argument is running up against the argument that it is the health-care system that needs to learn to be responsible. This is an argument that the Institute of Medicine put forth in a report that was issued in 2012 titled "Best Care at Lower Cost: The Path to Continuously Learning Health Care in America." The lead authors argue that this path requires that "research organizations, advocacy organizations, professional specialty societies, and care delivery organizations should facilitate the development, accessibility, and use of evidence-based and harmonized clinical practice guidelines."[12] It's a call for truth by committee. Somehow, all the conflicts of interest that color medical education[13] and patient care today will be cast aside for the sake of the system.

Fatuous or not, this is a call that resonates with professional educators in the medical academy. Medical education has been seeking credibility as a discipline for a generation. Today, a few medical schools have departments of education, but all have professionals on board dedicated to the implementation and analysis of preclinical and clinical education. Many years ago, a dear friend, one of the pioneers in the federal Department of Education, pointed out that schools of education were producing doctoral-level educators who would go unemployed were it not for the fact that schools of medicine were wedded to the notion that competence at the student level can be quantified in a fashion that is predictive of postgraduate, professional competence. Many schools have tweaked the Flexnerian curriculum with this goal in mind, proving yet again the old aphorism that most experiments in education are doomed to succeed for the first few years. It's not clear that any "experiment" in undergraduate pedagogy associates with improvement in the practice of medicine in the decades following graduation. The same pertains to formal postgraduate educational programs.[14]

Attempting to Quantify Clinical Competence

It is difficult to "teach" or grade ethical behavior or to supplant peer review for appraising a physician's accomplishments at the bedside of the individual patient. It is difficult to quantify the experience of satisfaction in knowing one did as much as possible for a patient. But it is possible to model all of these attributes of life as a physician, as well as necessary to recognize when they are lacking. Furthermore, it is possible to make this modeling the centerpiece of professionalism throughout one's life in medicine. The individual is the responsible agent of health care.

But if this is not modeled, if it is the responsibility of the "system" to foster a therapeutic team, to regulate its activity, and to monitor its effectiveness by audit, professionalism will be history and medicine just another manufacturing industry. That's where education theory would take us, as described by the authors of a 2013 article in the *Journal of the American Medical Association*: "There is increasing recognition that medical education should be adapted to address the integration of the electronic medical record into medical practice."[15] The mantra of this approach to medical education emphasizes targets of learning beyond the individual person, each with its own analytics. It is argued that educational institutions themselves, health-care delivery teams, and health-care delivery systems are each distinctive targets for learning goals that are at least as important as the more-traditional goal of educating the individual practitioner. Furthermore, each goal requires specific analytics to quantify achievement. To that end, the American Board of Internal Medicine (ABIM) and the Accreditation Council for Graduate Medical Education (ACGME) convened a task force composed of residency program directors, experts in evaluation and quality, and representatives of "internal medicine stakeholder organizations." The task force was charged with creating a reporting structure that calibrates whether trainees meet "milestones to achieve competency" in internal medicine. It was a daunting task that started with the compilation of a list of 142 "observable, developmental milestones" that were thought to capture the progression of knowledge skills and attitudes that culminates in proficiency. The result is a compendium of goals and evaluation instruments that has the granularity that would warm the hearts of those who are wedded to the Electronic Health Record. This material is available online[16] and is summarized in a recent paper.[17] It is anticipated that the degree to which trainees meet these milestones will influence whether training programs are accredited in the future.

By way of illustration, there are curricular milestones and grading scales for the "systems-based practice" goals. The former include an understanding of the roles and services provided by local health-delivery systems and familiarity with the negotiations necessary to effect patient-centered care among multiple care providers. (That's a lot of jargon that will be rendered less obscure in the next chapter.) Figure 3 is the template for grading competency for systems-based practice.

There are similar schemes for other dimensions of competency. This is an exercise in reductio ad absurdum. There are many others in the behavioral sciences, scales and metrics that are attempting to capture elements of satisfaction with relationships, or with working, and the like. Seldom is anything learned that could not be captured with a global score. That is the time-tested approach to assessing the competency of medical students and residents (and other work venues). When clinical training involved close interactions over time between individuals of varying experience, from medical students to attendings, consensus was reached and evaluations offered in a narrative format during the course of the interactions. Trainees were offered feedback in real time, so that any summary evaluation came as

11. Transitions patients effectively within and across health delivery systems. (SBP4)				
Critical Deficiencies			**Ready for unsupervised practice**	**Aspirational**
Disregards need for communication at time of transition Does not respond to requests of caregivers in other delivery systems	Inconsistently utilizes available resources to coordinate and ensure safe and effective patient care within and across delivery systems Written and verbal care plans during times of transition are incomplete or absent Inefficient transitions of care lead to unnecessary expense or risk to a patient (e.g. duplication of tests readmission)	Recognizes the importance of communication during times of transition Communication with future caregivers is present but with lapses in pertinent or timely information	Appropriately utilizes available resources to coordinate care and ensures safe and effective patient care within and across delivery systems Proactively communicates with past and future care givers to ensure continuity of care	Coordinates care within and across health delivery systems to optimize patient safety, increase efficiency and ensure high quality patient outcomes Anticipates needs of patient, caregivers and future care providers and takes appropriate steps to address those needs Role models and teaches effective transitions of care
☐ ☐	☐ ☐	☐ ☐	☐ ☐	☐
Comments:				

Systems-based Practice
The resident is demonstrating satisfactory development of the knowledge, skill, and attitudes/behaviors needed to advance in training. He/she is demonstrating a learning trajectory that anticipates the achievement of competency for unsupervised practice that includes the delivery of safe, effective, patient-centered, timely, efficient and equitable care.
_____ Yes _____ No _____ Conditional on Improvement

FIGURE 3 A template for grading the "competency" of medical trainees in "systems-based practice." (© 2012, the Accreditation Council for Graduate Medical Education and the American Board of Internal Medicine. All rights reserved.)

no surprise, including the summary evaluations represented by letters of recommendation.

The same reductionism in the name of granularity that is imposed on treatment acts by the Electronic Health Record[18] is now imposed on the educational process. And it doesn't stop with postgraduate training and board certification: the Continuing Medical Education (CME) industry discussed in chapter 3 welcomed with open coffers the notion that competence can be quantified. All sorts of certifying organizations are now selling continuing education programs that are designed to prepare practitioners for periodic examinations that are required for "maintenance of certification" (MOC). There is much consternation and some protest because of the costliness of these MOC agendas, costliness both in financial outlay (thousands of dollars) and time. Of course, the consternation and the protests would be inappropriate if the educational agenda was effective. As with much of modern reform, such as duty-hour restriction, the agenda is based on theory and promoted by those who claim special insights that merit both compliance

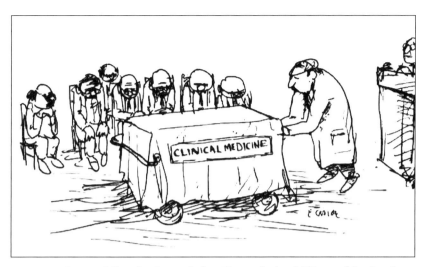

FIGURE 4 I was privileged to know the late Ernest Craige, M.D., as a friend and colleague on the faculty of the University of North Carolina for many decades. Ernie was a truly distinguished North Carolinian. He was the scion of a family that traced its roots in North Carolina to colonial times. His distinguished undergraduate career at UNC earned him a Rhodes Scholarship, after which he matriculated for an M.D. at Harvard and trained in medicine and cardiology at the Massachusetts General Hospital. He was one of several cardiologists to have been mentored by the legendary Paul Dudley White and carried the tradition of clinical acuity, compassion, and perspective with him throughout his life. In the mid-1950s, the legislature of North Carolina decided to turn its medical school into a four-year institution that granted the M.D. degree and build North Carolina Memorial Hospital as its teaching hospital. Ernie Craige was enticed back home as the founding chief of cardiology. He was a legendary educator, an exemplary physician and a renowned clinical scientist instrumental in the development of echocardiography. He was also an excellent artist and a brilliant cartoonist. His cartoons found their way into many a medical publication, *Pharos* in particular (as acknowledged in a special section of the February 1982 issue).

For years, we sat side by side at medical Grand Rounds. We whispered to each other about the content of presentations. Ernie was wont to turn to the blank side of the handout and draw cartoons about the theme of the presentation. Many were gifts to me. This is one. It was reproduced to illustrate an essay I wrote in *Clinical Research*, the journal of the American Federation for Clinical Research (Nortin M. Hadler, "De Morte Medicine," *Clinical Research* 32, no. 9 [1984]: 12). Both the journal and the federation are history.

and financial reward. However, the consternation and protest is anything but inappropriate. Attempts to show that these MOC agendas improve the quality of care or lower the costliness of care demonstrate just the opposite.[19]

When will "medical educators" realize that medical education continues throughout life and that competency is not a passing grade but a permanent goal? There is no scoring system that will substitute for peer review under the banner of professionalism. This reductionistic mindset may be the most iatrogenic sophism in the checkered history of caring for the patient. I have no doubt that it will be short-lived, though it has yet to approach full cycle.

CHAPTER EIGHT

Where Have All the Physicians Gone?

The seas are rising, the sands are shifting, and the pilings are no longer reliable. So it is with the American health-care system. Not long before I started to write this book, I declared, "Today, health is a commodity, disease is a product line, and physicians are a sales force in the employ of a predatory enterprise."[1] By the time I was drafting chapter 4, that sentiment had transformed to "patients became units of care, diseases became product lines, and physicians became production workers." By the time I completed the manuscript, patients were encounters, diseases were codes, doctors had been absorbed into the process of throughput, and the profession of medicine was wandering in "The Waste Land," "mixing memory and desire."

These are the unintended consequences of the evolution of the notion of "health" over the past fifty years. They are unintended, but long predictable. The mindset that believed it a good idea to reduce one of the most human of conditions, the experience of illness, to elemental components is now under the gun. The goal of capturing these elements in binary code has proved costly rather than cost saving. Serving the granularity of this exercise in reductionism has proved a task of such great complexity that any possibility of efficiency for patient care is sorely compromised. Defining efficiency as the care given per patient per unit of time demands an assembly line. Rewarding efficiency on this basis turns the reasoning into a tautology; moving patients through the delivery system more efficiently must be a good thing since it leads to more financial rewards.

It is remarkable how quickly this mindset has become entrenched. All sorts of new stakeholders were born and soon made room for any of the veteran stakeholders to climb aboard with barely a shibboleth, some murmuring "granularity" or "throughput" or "return on investment." There are the Invoice Mongers and their handmaidens: the coders, the auditors, the IT mavens purveying various iterations of the Electronic Health Record, and the consultants who profit from sprinkling serial heuristics on successive flaws in the software. There are the Quality Mongers who trumpet success by measuring outcome frequency, sometimes the frequency of adverse outcomes but seldom the frequency of clinically meaningful benefits; if "health care" is done well, efficiently, and paper free, why be concerned if it's useless? That's why when the number of patients whose HBA1c, blood pressure, or cholesterol is lowered, it is cause for elation on the part of these policy experts—but seldom on the part of patients, who are unlikely to experience more than the adverse effects of their compliance. Of course, the Quality Mongers are sophists because they rely on the Evidence Torturers to define Quality. These are responsible for the surreptitious corruption that plagues evidence-based medicine[2]—the misinterpretations, the hawking of small and irreproducible effects, the downplaying and hiding of results that are untoward from either the patient's or purveyor's perspectives, and the dominance of profits over ethics.

Much in the earlier chapters paints a dismal, even lurid picture of the evolution of the health-care system from a cottage industry to a conglomerate of patient-care assembly lines. We dissected how the "hospital" came to do a better job of sterilizing its intellectual atmosphere than its microbial pathogens, how caring professionals came to be time-clocked providers who are marching lockstep to the tunes played by a bloated, overpaid administration wedded to a flawed approach to optimizing cash flow. The result is a nation peppered with lumbering, costly, self-serving institutions that are playing a small role in fostering public welfare and a large role in rifling the public coffers. They are ethically bankrupt, highly leveraged houses of cards.

Everyone is standing back and scratching their heads, even those few who are amazed at the windfall this course of events has brought them. The body politic is consumed by an exercise in blame, in "I told you so" versus a torturing of the data in defense of the current approach. It is not at all clear that anyone is doing more than this, such as stepping back from the fray long enough to establish firm objectives, and strategies for when the objectives are not met in a timely fashion. Rather, it is not clear that the right hand knows what the left hand is doing, other than casting aspersions. As a result, all that is surfacing are excuses for the escalating costs shouldered by the "system," particularly by the individuals it is to serve, and the difficulty in demonstrating that increasing indemnification has resulted in something one might consider improved health. Furthermore, if there are advocates for the system who are working in the system, they are sotto voce. Work dissatisfaction, early retirement, elimination of discretionary budget lines, and layoffs are an ever-more-prominent feature of the health-care industry.

A Rational Solution

Despite all this, the mindset of the health-policy wonks is holding steady. Part of this intransigence is laudable; after all, it is inexcusable that the United States managed to hold off universal access to health care for a century longer than its sister advantaged countries. I fervently agree that this is now an unalienable right. However, that right is to *rational* health care, not to medicalization, overtreatment, overpricing, or iatrogenicity.

"The Morning Prayer of the Physician" is the legacy from antiquity for the tenets that would render health care rational. That prayer is draped in metaphysical allusions, however, and suffers from a degree of self-importance that sits poorly with me as well as with most contemporary ethicists. There is an update, a "prayer" offered by Sir Robert Hutchison in a letter to the editor of the *British Medical Journal* in March 1953. Hutchison was a Scottish physician and "paediatrician" who was long a professor at Great Ormond Street, the famous children's hospital in London. I learned of his legacy from several of the pediatric rheumatologists I worked with as a visiting scholar in London for two year in the 1970s. He was revered for his clinical acumen and remembered as a dour curmudgeon who seemed to enjoy tormenting his students by demonstrating their inadequacies. He wrote two textbooks; his *Clinical Methods* went through many editions and influenced two generations of British pediatricians. Sir Robert was a favorite of the British establishment, even to the extent of rising to be the 1st Baronet of Thurle. All of this aside, from my perspective, his major contribution was his "prayer":

> From inability to let well alone; from too much zeal for the new and contempt for what is old; from putting knowledge before wisdom, science before art, and cleverness before common sense, from treating patients as cases, and from making the cure of the disease more grievous than the endurance of the same, Good Lord, deliver us.

There are a number of approaches that would offer America a rational health-care system that would not violate either "The Morning Prayer" or Sir Robert's twentieth-century version. Furthermore, they would require per capita expenditures close to the average for the European Union rather than the multiples of that which make America an outlier from the perspective of the "health-care dollar" and a tragedy from the perspective of the benefit/cost ratio, the bang for the buck. I have been modeling such a rational system that targets overhead and overtreatment but not patient empowerment or the doctor-patient relationship. The next chapter details some of these efforts.

Overhead is easy to render transparent: why are we paying more for more management "support" than any other industry or country? Overtreatment is also easy to render transparent once one understands the basic principles of the philosophy of science. All science, including clinical science, is a valid way to reject any hypothesis; the "proof" of a hypothesis is always tentative. Hence, the "evidence" that makes medicine incontrovertibly "evidence based" is the evidence that rejects hypotheses. Testing for the clinically meaningful efficacy of drugs, devices, procedures, or policies is often feasible, and many results have been published. All these merit close inspection. When there is no compelling evidence for a clinically meaningful benefit, the hypothesis should be considered untenable, and underwriting must be withheld. That simple tenet is the other secret to rational health care.

The reason we cannot have a rational health-care system in the United States is the entropy in the current system that is purchased and nurtured by the deep pockets of its stakeholders. That was the lesson we learned in our attempt at piloting our innovative indemnity scheme a decade ago. That was also the nemesis of "Obamacare." Considerations of cost and costliness were "redlined" out of the final versions of the legislation by members of congressional committees whose opinions were swayed by health-care-industry lobbyists that prowl the halls of power, some six lobbyists for every member. We will not have a rational system until the public learns what to demand as rational and realizes that rational is not rationing. I am hoping the learning curve will escalate in the near future when the houses of cards start to fall apart, one by one, and the country opens its mind to new solutions. In fact, driving this learning curve is one of the principles of the approach we're taking. Furthermore, we're determined to preempt the chaos of the implosion of the current system—but I'm getting ahead of myself.

For now, we're stuck with the old mindset and the desperate attempts of the current crop of influential policy wonks to tweak "Obamacare" before universal access is sacrificed to the disappointments in which it is swimming. Much of the rollout and early challenges relate to the inpatient component of the health-care systems. Everything that the Affordable Care Act was to render affordable has yet to materialize in the inpatient setting. Attempts to reform the reforms in this regard are under way but are proving challenging to say the least. That has caused the policy experts to focus on decreasing the demand for inpatient care with the expectation that affordability will follow. To accomplish this reduction in hospitalizations, it seems reasonable to apply the same reductionistic approach to the outpatient setting that should have worked in the inpatient setting. Hence, putatively efficient systems are rolled out of the federal policy works bearing a dizzying array of acronyms and rolled into various models of outpatient management. This exercise has brought into the Department of Health and Human Services and its codependent consulting and academic constituency a growing corps of health-policy specialists who increasingly display their MBA more prominently than any other graduate credential they might have earned. The outpatient is an arena of health care reform that rapidly is catching up with the inpatient arena in confusion, inadequate documentation, dearth of scientific validation, and costliness.

Doctors' Offices

While the role of "inpatient" and the "hospital" in twenty-first-century America is a very far cry from what it was in the mid-twentieth century, the "outpatient" and the "office" have changed less dramatically. Through the 1950s, multispecialty and group practices were rare on the East Coast and looked down upon by organized medicine. To the East Coast establishment, the spate of group practices elsewhere were looked upon with suspicion—including the Mayo, Gunderson, Guthrie, and other clinics, as well as the Kaiser-Permanente conglomerate. The traditional solo private practitioner was quick to accuse such practices of the unethical practice of fee splitting, the overt or surreptitious practice of rewarding the referring doctor for the referral. Besides, multispecialty clinics in urban America were the stuff of charity care, below the dignity of the carriage trade.

By the 1960s, the solo private practitioner had come to realize the advantages of collective efforts, particularly the economies of scale in sharing facilities and staff and in common usage of laboratory and radiology and the "convenience" of reliable referral sources. With the advent of Medicare and the Blue Shields, clinics staffed by physicians practicing different specialties or the same specialty became commonplace. The physicians developed their own patient lists but shared support staff, rotated night and call coverage, and negotiated contracts as a business entity for common needs, such as health and liability insurance and pensions. Many owned their own building, often with a clinical laboratory and even a radiology suite. Surgical groups might add procedure rooms and a professional staff for postprocedure care, even rehabilitation. Usually, one of the physicians took on the managing role of these small corporations.

For decades, this was a highly successful business model. It was well matched to the demands of insured patients who came to expect a degree of personal comfort as outpatients that was a lesser priority for institutions invested and investing in inpatient care. These private clinics were also a match for the growth of governmental regulations aimed at maintaining patient safety and privacy and at assuring that ownership of profitable ancillary facilities was not an important determinant of the quantity of care. Despite federal regulations, the practice of "self-referral" remains several-fold more frequent than non-self-referral, particularly for imaging and anatomic pathology.[3]

Toward the end of the twentieth century, the multispecialty clinics started to come apart. This was largely a reflection of the disparities in reimbursement. Specialties that were entrenched in procedures, such as colonoscopies and various cardiac tests, were far more lucrative, bringing in revenues that supported the clinic and the specialist handsomely—much more handsomely than physicians whose practice did not include highly priced elements. The interventionalists came to feel that they were being tithed to support colleagues whose billing was relatively meager, a resentment that might not be fully assuaged by a differential in salary. That's the explanation for the proliferation of freestanding intervention centers, such as endoscopy centers, orthopedic clinics, heart clinics, and their kin. That leaves behind the "cognitive" practitioners who had to support the facility and their incomes with the income derived from taking care of patients rather than parts of patients. Their only fallback was in increasing "throughput" at a price of declining career satisfaction. These are the clinics that the marauding health-care systems are either buying up or, increasingly, simply outcompeting. These are the patients who are being swallowed up by the more-expensive coding systems of the health centers. These are the doctors who are retiring early or applying for employment at a lower but more reliable income in the health-care system.

As an aside, many of these retiring doctors are far from retiring in their desire to care for patients. Many are not strapped financially. Clinics started popping up a decade ago to serve the desires of these physicians to serve and the needs of the uninsured needy. It's a movement that has a growing presence (http://volunteersinmedicine.org/). It is successful in innumerable ways. These retired volunteer physicians are neither paid nor allowed to work more than a day or two a week. More important, they are allowed to design their own templates; they decide how many patients they will see and how much time they spend with each. The result is satisfied patients and satisfied doctors. The patients get the time to communicate their concerns, and the doctors have the time to listen and practice according to their conscience. Any reader who has health insurance would be better off in one of these clinics, but lack of insurance is a requirement. Eat your hearts out; if only the country realized that this is the secret to care and caring—and it can be supported on a meager budget. But the din of the health-care system drowns out the message. As a result, this is a drop in the bucket when it comes to the health of the nation, but it's a drop of pure water in a very muddy bucket.

Gatekeepers

Since the attempt to target hospital systems for the sake of affordability has been largely co-opted by the costliness of the approach and the ability of hospital systems to game the system, policy experts have been tweaking the latest versions of the multispecialty clinic, even though the lucrative specialties have fled and the more viable of these clinics have been purchased by various health-care systems. The policy approach is based on a simple tenet: if disease can be managed efficiently in the outpatient clinics, the need for recourse in hospitals would be abrogated and their costliness circumvented. This is the reasoning that is driving some of the reforms in Graduate Medical Education we discussed previously. In an amusing gambit, the policy experts decided there must be another designation for these clinics to distinguish their novelty and desirability:

- *Patient-Centered* is one shibboleth, as if this is a radical innovation. Clinics have always been patient-centered. As with hospitals, the issue is whether the patients are advantaged by being the center of attention.
- *Medical Homes* are another shibboleth, also touted as a radically new idea. However, it is really the idea embodied by the American "family practice" or, recently, the British "general practice," where a "team" is the primary caregiver from cradle to grave. Usually, a physician is designated the responsible cognitive leader working with the administrator responsible for infrastructure. As has been true for some time, the roles played by the members of the team are in flux. Some "medical homes" assign an "intake" nurse responsible for asking the patient what's wrong and directing him or her to what is presumed to be the person with the solution. Some larger "medical homes" have pharmacists, even pharmacists with a doctorate in pharmacy,

monitoring prescriptions. Some make use of nurse practitioners more than medical doctors as resources. And some designate a single practitioner to the care of each patient with rules for cross-coverage.

- *Accountable Care Organizations* (ACO) are the most ludicrous of the neologisms because all they denote is another attempt at the promulgation of a Health Maintenance Organization (HMO). An ACO is a patient-centered medical home that is capitated, meaning it is given a fixed sum of money based on the number of enrolled patients and charged with living within these means. The better the ACO lives within its means, the less the allocated sum of money is expended, leaving behind a "profit." In America, it is a viable model as long as the patients are not too sick and the means substantial. It is the business model for the Kaiser-Permanente organization. The Medicare administration is fostering ACOs around the country with the expectation that primary-care physicians can burden the "chief executive" function regarding expenditures and reimbursement while maintaining quality of care. Many in the policy world are applauding.[4] Of course, all are aware of the potential for perverse incentives in a capitated delivery model. Will care be withheld, or more expensive care withheld, to pad the pot at the end of the budgetary cycle? To do so overtly would be unethical, if not illegal, as the U.S. Veteran's Administration is demonstrating. However, how can we develop some assurance that such false efficiency is not a subliminal action?

- *Pay-for-Performance* is proposed as a solution to maintaining the quality of care in ACOs (and elsewhere). Obviously, in an ACO, there is an incentive to offer care so efficiently that there are residual funds to disburse to the members of the staff at the end of the budgetary cycle. It is not clear how many and how often ACOs are even able to stay within their budgets, let alone have a surplus. It isn't even clear how to distribute any surplus fairly among physicians, physician assistants, nurse practitioners, and others.[5] Should it be based on performance, or should some component or all be distributed regardless of performance in deference to a "team" spirit? If it's by performance, what weight should be given to experience, clinical purview, and patient mix (relative degree of clinical challenge)? And what do we mean by "performance"?

This last question is at the very heart of health care. What do we mean by "performance," and can we measure it in order to value it? These are neither trivial nor long-ignored questions. A decade ago, the "Quality and Outcomes Framework" was introduced in the United Kingdom. General practitioners are essentially salaried, but this framework tied a quarter of their income to measures of performance. It also provided a wealth of data that has provided fodder for waves of British number crunchers and the basis for a great many publications. The 2004 version of the framework detailed a great number of performance indicators: clinical indicators (the likes of blood pressure control or unanticipated hospitalizations), organizational indicators (record keeping, training programs, and the like) and patient experience indicators (various satisfaction surveys). It sounds sensible, but the analyses produced disquieting results. The income incentives did alter physician behavior, but they increasingly were seen by physicians as a "distraction, diverting their gaze onto limited parts of clinical practice and reducing the focus on the patient's agenda during the consultation."[6] After a decade of tweaking the framework, major changes were recently instituted, such as placing less income at risk and trying to develop more meaningful indicators, such as proactive management of the vulnerable elderly patient. The Quality and Outcomes Framework is moving away from its love of granularity to incentivize professionalism. It is trying to extricate humanism from the flood of metrics.[7]

But far be it from the American policy experts to learn from the experience of others. After all, we are Americans, and we can succeed past where others have strived. And if at first we don't succeed, "try again" is the rallying call, rather than "back to the drawing board." We are, however, having trouble succeeding in our initial attempts. Take as an example the Pennsylvania Chronic Care Initiative, a pilot of a multipayer medical home that introduced a series of quality initiatives and offered a considerable financial incentive if the practices complied.[8] A cadre of scientists from the Rand Corporation and other prestigious policy think tanks did their best to parse out some good news—and failed. There was no reduction in utilization of hospitals,

Emergency Departments, or outpatient care services, and therefore no cost savings, over the course of three years. There was also no improvement in the quality-of-care indicators that were followed, with the exception of a slight increase in screening for one of the complications of diabetes.

I have no doubt that the systems approach will remain a sacred cow for some time. It has commandeered inpatient facilities to the point of bankruptcy. Rather than abandon the approach, good money is sent after bad in the belief that the basic idea is valid. And the systems perspective is rapidly coming to commandeer outpatient care. The early disappointments are discounted as demonstrations of errors in design, or in target population, or in both,[9] rather than errors in concept. The call in the halls of power is to take this failing concept to new heights and create a new category of provider under Medicare, an "Advanced Primary Care Practice" (APCP), with a new payment model. Care management fees would "flow on behalf of a defined population in a predictable way, incorporating accountability for population health outcomes and opportunities for shared savings."[10]

The Master Clinician

We've covered decades of notions of health and the responses of medicine to caring for people when health is lacking. We started out in the introduction with some of the attempts of the leading thinkers at the beginning of the twentieth century to cast medicine as a caring profession with a humanistic calling and a scientific foundation. That was a time when little else mattered more, and in retrospect, little else was effective until the postwar era dawned. We then wandered through the heady times when science was productive and relevant, so that treating the patient took a backseat to treating the patient's disease. We watched as this era was corrupted by overtreatment, fostered first by hubris and later by profit motives. The country did not recognize this tendency as wrong, let alone evil, and it still doesn't. But affordability and escalating costs are handmaidens that are ever more difficult to ignore. The response is to view medicine as an industry that should be amenable to maneuvers that have been a match for issues in affordability and cost in other industries. All we have to do is fix the system so as to eliminate inefficiencies while maintaining quality. That mantra has backfired and is backfiring dramatically from a fiscal perspective. Soon it will play out from an institutional perspective, probably inelegantly.

It is already playing out tragically from the perspective of those who are ill and those who really care about them. Two physicians bear witness. These were giants and pioneers in their medical disciplines. Both recently shared personal stories, painful stories, of their experiences with the suffering of illness in the current institution of medicine. Arthur Kleinman, a Harvard psychiatrist and pioneer in medical anthropology, describes living with his wife's terminal dementia in an essay titled "From Illness as Culture to Caregiving as Moral Experience."[11] The late Arnold (Bud) Relman had a distinguished career plied in many venues, from the chair of medicine at the University of Pennsylvania to editor in chief of the *New England Journal of Medicine*. He cast his wise and wizened eyes on the comings and goings around his bed in the Intensive Care Unit of Massachusetts General Hospital, where he had to remain for months in order to survive fracturing his neck.[12] Both Dr. Kleinman and Dr. Relman explain how the system, the technology, and the science were themselves inadequate. Both speak about the people involved in the giving of care as crucial. I'm not sure either would have imagined arriving at such a conclusion when they were at the peak of their careers some thirty years ago.

Many others will come to this realization. When they do, we will have come full circle and returned to the ideal of medical humanism described in the introduction. For now, we will have to settle for those few voices, like mine, that expect to be heard but don't expect to be listened to. We don't need carrots and sticks to incentivize caring; that approach has been tested, and it doesn't work. We don't need a highly efficient production line that moves units of care through the factory of "health care" and out the back profitably; that approach has been tested, and it doesn't work either. We don't need to shorten medical school; what you can teach quickly and learn superficially is only the start to maturing as a physician. There are only shortcuts to doing things *to* patients, not doing things *for* patients.

What we desperately need are ethical physician incentives and a shared purpose in the sense that Max Weber, the great pioneer in sociology, described a century ago.[13] We want to inculcate into medical students the notion that the practice of medicine is a privilege, a responsibility, a high calling, and a ministry. We need to build peer review into the way we approach the bedside, not for the sake of quality control but for the sake of quality enhancement. We want the aspiration to be a master clinician to be the rule, even among those whose talents fall short or are co-opted in part by acquiring less cognitive skills.

Beyond nurturing a body of knowledge and honing clinical skills, the master clinician takes to heart the teachings of the likes of Martin Buber in *The Knowledge of Man*:

> Man wishes to be confirmed in his being by man,
> And wishes to have a presence in the being of the other . . .
> Secretly and bashfully he watches for a YES which allows him to be
> And which can come only from one human person to another.

I firmly believe that there are many physicians who share this creed but find it impossible to live by it given the constraints imposed by the current health-care delivery system. Furthermore, nearly all attempts to reform this system represent little more than a slight trim for Medusa. It would be wonderful if we could start anew, but we missed that opportunity in 1912 when the platform of the Progressive Party was relegated to history with the defeat of Theodore Roosevelt's second bid for the presidency of the country. That platform called for a national health insurance scheme. We could wait for the current health-care delivery system to implode and hope that a new way forward will be apparent to all when (if) the dust settles.

Or we could see our way clear to overlay the current system with a structure that offers patients and physicians a path to rational health care. That is no mean task, given the chaos of the current system. Every stakeholder speaks of reform but only gets enthusiastic when the reform targets another category of stakeholder or is designed in a fashion that represents a minor threat to the profitability of his or her stake. That is one of the flaws of the Affordable Care Act. But it is the fate of any attempt to reform the U.S. health-care system head-on. I can attest to that futility from personal experience with legislative reform, not just as a student of policy.

The only possibility is to find a way around the wall of self-interest that surrounds American health care. In the next chapter, I explain the background and operational details of one such way. However, any reform must occur on the moral high ground in order to be sustainable. Health care must not place the care of the patient and nurturing of the patient-physician dialogue at the center of the "system"; health care *is* the care of the patient and the nurturing of the patient-physician dialogue. The "system" is infrastructure.

CHAPTER NINE

Medical Professionalism in the Twenty-First Century

It is one thing to champion a trustworthy patient-physician relationship that promotes informed medical decision making and proclaim the physician to be the wise facilitator in such a relationship. But it is quite another thing to extricate such a relationship from the current dialectic, which is heavily funded to promote a systems approach to patient care. I find it impossible to remain passive in the face of this dialectic. There is an old proverb in medical circles that internists know everything but do nothing, and surgeons know nothing yet do everything. I am an internist. But I am a loose-cannon internist.

There is a desperate need to position the patient's narrative as raison d'être and a desperate need to provide wise ears to hear it. The only way that will happen is to create an atmosphere that demands it, an administrative structure that supports it, and a reimbursement scheme based on fees for serving. Getting there is an uphill battle, somewhat Sisyphean given the powerful push-back from stakeholders in the status quo, but it is not insurmountable. The top of the hill is the moral high ground. Medical professionalism must plant its flag there because there is no other way to serve patients well in the twenty-first century.

Finding a way to plant that flag has been a twenty-five-year odyssey for me, but it has not been a steady upward climb. In fact, it was a gentle saunter for many years because there was neither urgency nor an obvious path of least resistance. Besides, these were years when I was focused on my career as an educator and clinical investigator while American medicine was reveling in its transformation into a behemoth. It was difficult to step aside long enough to effectively question the enthusiasm surrounding me. It became less difficult when I realized that the aspects of my career and my competence that I valued the most were losing value in the new version of American medicine. I felt little pain since other aspects of my career were thriving, but colleagues who were focusing exclusively on the bedside found themselves progressively disenfranchised. So about fifteen years ago, I started to climb with more determination. It was clear that the developing version of American medicine was no champion of my notion of excellence at the bedside. It was clear that prior versions of American medicine had too many flaws to bemoan their passing. And it was clear that American realpolitik would not countenance a national health-insurance scheme, not even the copying of elements of such schemes that were successful elsewhere. The hope was in finding a way to overlay the American approach with a layer of rationality and reestablish the patient-physician relationship at the center of American medicine. That would require figuring out a way to monetize altruism.

Health Assurance, Disease Insurance

A decade ago, I described an approach to "health-care" insurance that I call the health assurance–disease insurance scheme.[1] This is designed as a benefit that can be provided to workers by employers or to citizens by state governments. It is meant as a rational alternative to the current systems of employer-sponsored health insurance. The approach takes advantage of a science that explores salutary options and rejects those that are ineffective or harmful.

My proposal has two novel features. First, it is a "defined contribution" plan rather than the customary "defined benefit" plan. This means that a fixed amount of money is allocated each year, calculated as a percentage of wages or as an income tax, for the purpose of covering health-care costs. The challenge is to provide the benefit within these fiscal limitations. The traditional "defined benefit" scheme calls for paying for all or some of whatever health plan is offered; the challenge is to debate which plan is affordable, or affordable with or without a contribution from the indemnified in terms of deductibles, co-pays, or both.

One might imagine that both schemes would arrive at the same goal for the same cost, but that's naïve. The defined benefit places most control in the hands of the purveyors and administrators of health care, with little need for efficiency. It's more of a "this is what we're selling; you need to figure out a way to buy it." In practice, it's even more perverse than that since the purveyors of a defined benefit plan (such as Cigna or Blue Cross) charge an administrative fee, a negotiated percentage of the river of money flowing through the system from the paying employer to the paid provider. There is no incentive to restrict the flow and little way for the payer to cry foul as the river heads toward flood level. Crying foul runs into accusations of "rationing" and can invoke the wrath of ERISA, the Employee Retirement Income Security Act passed by Congress in 1974 to give participants the right to sue for benefits if the management of a benefits plan breaches fiduciary duty. The rise in health-care expenditures in America would not be outstripping all sister countries were it not for these leaking floodgates. Despite an outlay that now exceeds $3 trillion annually, it has not been possible to demonstrate that the American citizenry is more advantaged in terms of health and longevity than the citizens of sister nations that expend a fraction of the amount per capita. In 2013 the National Academies Press published "Best Care at Lower Cost," a report of a committee of the Institute of Medicine that was charged, in part, with an analysis of this discordance. It was estimated that about a third of America's health-care expenditure supports excessive administration, overpricing, and clinically inappropriate care.[2] Examples of clinically inappropriate care include interventions that are ineffective, unnecessary, harmful, or overlooked.

The defined contribution scheme that I proposed places a mandate on the management of the plan to live within the budget. This advantages the payer in that cost is predictable and up front. But it advantages the participant only to the extent that "rationing" is not unleashed. Rationing is meant to imply withholding clinically meaningful care for any reason. It does not imply withholding care that is not clinically meaningful; that would be rational. Debates over rationing versus rational have played out in court under the ERISA statute, where the discussion of the relevant science is colored by the pathos of clinical realities. It's difficult to hear of a terrible outcome without assuming to some degree that the "rationed" intervention would have made a difference, despite a science to the contrary. This dialectic plays out infrequently in the realm of the defined benefit plans, which are rewarded for circumventing litigation by simply providing the unproved and the unprovable. This is a profitable fallback for a defined benefit plan, but it is the Achilles heel for a defined contribution plan.

The second novel feature of the health assurance–disease insurance scheme is that the money resulting from the defined contribution is allocated to two separate funds: a disease insurance fund and a health assurance fund. The former is a shared risk pool that underwrites most medical care except that for which no clinically meaningful benefit is demonstrable in systematic, scientific studies. Shared risk is the concept that underlies all insurance; a population buys the policy to insure that any individual among them who faces a loss will not suffer unbearable consequences. The health assurance fund is not a shared risk pool. It accumulates all moneys from the defined contribution that are not expended for disease insurance. This health assurance pool of money is available on a pro rata basis for any health-related intervention that is not covered by disease insurance but is licensed for purveyance in the participant's state. This could run a gamut from naturopathic interventions that are licensed in some states to chiropractic interventions that are licensed in all states. It could also include medical interventions that are licensed but are not covered by disease insurance because the supporting science is not convincing. Or it might be expended on interventions that are not purported to be disease specific but are supported as salutary by scientific studies, interventions such as job retraining, English as a second language, and marriage counseling. Such services should be provided because a rational approach calls for treating the whole patient, and improved employment prospects and domestic contentment benefit one's health and quality of life.

Pivotal in the administration of the health assurance–disease insurance scheme is the definition of effectiveness. The design calls for the establishment of "Clinimetrics Units." The term "Clinimetrics" was coined by the late Alvan Feinstein and was the title of one of his books.[3] Feinstein started his career as a cardiologist when he saw the need to apply a critical and quantitative razor to the rationale for all clinical interventions. He became a pioneer in the evidence-based medicine (EBM) movement, an outspoken advocate for rational health care, and a man with whom I enjoyed many memorable discussions. The

Clinimetrics Unit would be staffed by physicians trained in the statistical and epidemiological methods required to evaluate evidence. They would be an independent agency that would maintain a firm distance from potentially conflictual relationships. Their task was to evaluate the available science to generate determinations of the effectiveness of particular medical and surgical interventions. These determinations would inform coverage under the disease insurance fund.

A Workers' Compensation Epiphany

This is only a brief overview of the health assurance–disease insurance scheme. It is a defined contribution scheme that places the patient at its center; it has a fiduciary role to underwrite effective care for its participants in such a fashion that money saved reverts to the participant for health-related discretionary spending. There is much more detail and econometric modeling to describe, but that would be useful only as an exercise in historical inquiry. Shortly after the new millennium had begun, I presented the scheme to a sizable group of stakeholders in one of the few states that countenances any innovation in their statutes that define the regulation of health insurance. I offered the scheme solely as a solution for the uninsured worker, generally part-time employees or employees of small businesses that could not afford to offer a health-care benefit. Counted among the stakeholders in attendance were executives from insurance companies offering defined benefit plans, executives from large corporations, and state officers. The audience was rapt, the reception was polite—and the scheme was sidelined.

I learned valuable lessons in realpolitik. It was clear that for many reasons, from familiarity to greed, there was little room to superimpose rationality on America's state-by-state system of employer-sponsored, defined benefit health insurance. The push-back was powerful and well-funded then, and it remains so to this day. Of all the programmatic vulnerabilities built into the Affordable Care Act by dint of political bludgeoning, the reliance on a defined benefit model and the expurgation of any language demanding *cost*-effectiveness may prove the most telling.

At about the same time I was having my comeuppance, I had an epiphany. Perhaps driven by my notion of a communitarian ethic,[4] the epiphany came under the rubric "workers' compensation insurance." I have been a student of workers' compensation indemnity schemes for nearly forty years. That has caused me to become familiar with many literatures and mind-sets that are generally considered to be a long way from clinical purview. My goal was not to gain expertise in labor economics, risk management, labor relations and regulations, ergonometrics, or the details and history of social legislation. Rather, I explored all these disciplines with the goal of understanding and dissecting constraints that the sociopolitical process places on clinical decision making in America and a dozen other countries. More than a hundred research papers and many academic editorials, chapters, and books bear witness to these efforts.[5]

A brief history demonstrates the necessity of understanding how we can bend the notion of "workers' compensation insurance" to serve the goal of superimposing rationality on the American approach to providing health insurance by dragging the patient-doctor relationship to center stage. "Workmen's compensation insurance" was the only facet of European social welfare legislation to make landfall in the United States in the early twentieth century, and it was not an easy trip. New York passed its workers' compensation law in 1910, but the U.S. Supreme Court declared it unconstitutional. At the time, the Court interpreted the Commerce Clause of the U.S. Constitution to prohibit state laws that regulate interstate commerce. Congress passed statutes providing workers' compensation for federal employees, railroad workers, and others involved in interstate commerce. New York's statute reemerged in 1913. New Jersey's statute was enacted in 1911, and others followed state by state over the next decades; Mississippi passed its law after World War II. (This is the precedent for each state legislating health insurance when it came to that at midcentury.) There are important differences in administration and regulation of workers' compensation insurance schemes across the states, but all share a basic premise: any worker who suffers a personal injury that arises out of or in the course of working is provided whatever medical and surgical recourse is available to make him or her whole again and sufficient financial compensation so that there is no loss in wages while under treatment. Once it is decided that further improvement is unlikely, work capacity is assessed. If wage-earning capacity is compromised, workers' compensation insurance provides financial compensation to make up for the likely loss in wages. Unique to the American workers' compensation system is a compromise that was struck at the time of the earliest state legislation: management support was contingent on including "tort immunity" in the legislation. That means, short of malfeasance, the injured worker cannot sue the employer. Hence, workers' compensation is excluded from ERISA.

Workers' compensation claims that involve violent events and traumatic outcomes were the primary consideration early in the century. As "occupational diseases" were recognized—diseases such as those resulting from toxic chemical exposures at work—amendments were written to provide recourse. To this day, recourse for these categories of work-related illnesses is generally considered a triumph of social legislation; treatment from a medical and monetary perspective is efficient and cost-effective. Furthermore, there are parallel pressures to prevent injuries in the first place. The premiums charged to employers are adjusted by "experience rating" of the job categories; more injuries lead to higher premiums. And regulatory statutes and agencies came into being to promote safe work environments and penalize employers for falling short.

In the 1930s, a wrinkle was introduced to the workers' compensation system. Harvard surgeons ascribed back pain to herniation of the disc and went so far as to label the illness a "rupture." Workers' compensation venues were already challenged with discerning whether particular conditions, such as "telegraphist's wrist," qualified as having risen out of or in the course of employment. Backache did not enter the debate until it was ascribed to a ruptured disc. After all, it was argued, if the outcome is so violent as to be considered a "rupture," the inciting event need not be extraordinary to consider the back pain an injury and therefore compensable. It followed that any task that made the back pain more intense should be assumed to be the task that caused the back to hurt in the first place. Furthermore, workers' compensation should underwrite any and all interventions that are offered as solutions to the worker's disabling back "injury," unleashing surgical zeal and hubris, a flood of prescription opiates, the flowering of ergonomics, and an epidemic of disabling chronic back pain even in industries where tasks are progressively less physically demanding.

The social construction of the "injured back" was a sea change for the administration of workers' compensation schemes around the world. Today, about 80 percent of the cost of workers' compensation insurance relates to low back pain and similar regional musculoskeletal disorders. It also was a sea change in the common sense regarding these disorders. For some time, I have argued that a worker whose back pain is branded an injury is at great risk of iatrogenic outcomes ranging from unnecessary procedures and drugs to wandering forlorn in the Kafka-esque world of disability determination. A policy that works so well on behalf of a worker who has suffered an amputation, laceration, burn, or the like can turn evil when the same policy poultice is applied to illness experiences that are not peculiar to the workplace. I argued that it was irrational and harmful.

Then along came my epiphany. Why not embrace this irrationality, push it to its logical end, and mold it to the service of the American worker who is ill from *any* cause? All of us can countenance calling a backache an "injury." What reasonable hindrance is there to calling a headache an injury as well? And what about an upper respiratory illness? It probably is work related; it is caused by viruses in exhaled droplets, and we have more exposure to such at work than most other places we visit each day. (By the way, if one chooses to label an inguinal hernia in a worker as a "rupture," it is compensable, too.)

Twenty-Four-Hour Coverage

So, if a backache can be declared an injury, why not a headache, or a heart attack, or pneumonia, or . . .

Does this seem fatuous? I would argue that it is no more fatuous than labeling a backache an injury. If some physical predicaments can be redefined, many others can be as well, and consequently, the worker can be covered for all morbid events twenty-four hours a day and not just for accidental injuries in the course of working.

This line of reasoning moves health insurance for the worker under the workers' compensation umbrella. It is not an entirely novel idea. Why should a worker be forced to turn to particular doctors and forms of care on the basis of insurance rather than on the basis of the particular illness? California ran a pilot twenty-four-hour coverage scheme in the early 1990s (Labor Code Section 4612), which supported workers' choosing a provider rather than being forced to seek care for an "injury" only from a provider designated by their workers' compensation carrier. The results were difficult to interpret, in part because the economy and labor force were in flux, but the twenty-four-hour-coverage notion did stir enthusiasm for a while. Some of its advocates were seeking the cost shifting from workers' compensation coffers to health-insurance coffers. Some were aware of the discordance in customary treatment; for example, workers' compensation claimants with backache were far more likely to be afforded surgery and opiates than similar individuals who sought care from physicians reimbursed under health-insurance policies. Despite favorable policy considerations,[6] both the policy and the tendency to try innovations eventually faded into obscurity.

Nevertheless, there are obvious advantages to the twenty-four-hour scheme. First, it removes the requirement of work relatedness from access to care. There no longer is a distinction between caring for the insured worker if there is or is not a causal relationship between the illness and exposures at work. Care should be designed solely to benefit the patient and not be tailored to the claimant. And it removes issues in disability determination and compensability from the encounter between a patient and the treating clinician. They are important, but quite separate exercises; combining them compromises both in a way that does a disservice to the patient. Disability determination and compensability are much more regulatory than clinical constructs; they need a separate venue.

Finally, the history, politics, legislation, regulation, advocacy, actuarial science, econometrics, and much else that supports the workers' compensation establishment has developed in parallel with all that supports the health-insurance establishment in America. Seldom do the twain meet, or know much in depth about the other, for that matter. Even my colleagues in the august National Academy of Social Insurance are largely stratified along these lines. The stakeholders in one would be ill-prepared to defend against the incursions of the other, although these are quick studies when it comes to their business turf. This means that bringing health care under the workers' compensation umbrella is less likely to run into resistance from an entrenched bureaucracy guarding its turf.

Universal Workers' Compensation Insurance

Now let's see what happens if we impose the defined contribution, health assurance–disease insurance model on a twenty-four-hour workers' compensation scheme in one of the states. Rather than calling this twenty-four-hour coverage, the rubric is now Universal Workers' Compensation Insurance (UWCI).

There are several states where the legislation establishing the workers' compensation insurance scheme offers some room for innovation. There are even several states that have legislated "opt out," the option to offer a designer policy in exchange for relinquishing tort immunity. Nonetheless, any attempt to introduce a Universal Workers' Compensation Act (UWCA) would require innovative legislation, and any carrier of UWCI would need an equally innovative approach to management and finances. For example, the fiduciary principle for the expenditure of the defined contribution funds remains, but instead of pro rata contributions to their individual health assurance fund, the participants will receive their equal portion of unspent money as an annual share (that portion of the unspent money allocated to the individual employee). This share can be used only to purchase one of several supplemental policies ("wraps"), all related to their health and welfare. UWCI does not cover obstetrics, for example, but there is an obstetrical wrap. One might prefer a health savings account (HSA), but equitable administration would be prohibitive given the structure of the UWCI program and the mobility of the American workforce.

The premium charged to the employee in a UWCI program should be a small percentage of salary, the same percentage across the entire salary range, with the employer matching the aggregate contribution by a multiple of two. For the employee, this means the CEO might be paying a percent or two of millions of dollars, while the entry-level worker is paying a percent or two of thousands. There is no co-pay or deductible provision, nor is an employee excluded for prior medical conditions. This is a progressive form of a fixed-contribution benefit that provides a considerable war chest for a UWCI carrier to exercise its fiduciary role, particularly since profitability is not the primary goal and is limited in the UWCA. That means there is a mandate to minimize overhead, negotiate the cost of interventions that are overpriced, and eschew the ineffective.

Realize that most labor-intensive companies are forced to monitor their personnel costs closely. A major component of these costs is employee benefits. For that reason, it is common for these companies to meet their labor needs with part-time workers and thereby avoid offering benefits that can vary in cost unpredictably. Major companies have been forced into bankruptcy by such a toll, companies such as Kmart and Sears. The UWCI premium is fixed, predictable, and far less burdensome than either current workers' compensation or health-insurance premiums. These advantages almost certainly will make it feasible for corporations to transition from part-time employment to a full-time workforce. Labor and management benefit from the UWCA. Only stakeholders profiting from the current health-care system will be hurt.

These and many more of the administrative and financial details are crucial and fascinating. My intent in this chapter is to offer a way out of the cul-de-sac that has come to entrap the American patient-physician relationship, and the UWCA provides the solution in the way it informs the limits of clinical certainty and incentivizes rational care. It is a solution that can set the precedent for underwriting the provision of rational care for generations to come. It is worthy of close consideration. It is the foundation for an enlightened patient-doctor relationship.

Clinically Meaningful Interventions

The legislation that establishes a UWCI also establishes a separate and independent Clinical Effectiveness Panel (CEP). The CEP is charged with a role similar to that of the "Clinimetrics Unit" in the health assurance–disease insurance scheme. The UWCA specifies that the deliberations of this panel are privileged, and that neither the panel nor its individual members can be sued. Hence, the CEP enjoys a level of exclusivity in their activities akin to a state supreme court. Legal recourse is available under the Universal Workers' Compensation Act, but it embroils the insurance companies who choose to take advantage of the determinations of the CEP.

CEP membership consists of six medical doctors and three attorneys. All are chosen from a pool of senior professionals with considerable academic credentials and accomplishments. All must be free of conflictual ties, financial or otherwise, to any of the stakeholders whose activities might be perturbed by determinations emanating from the CEP. The medical doctors, furthermore, must have considerable clinical experience and must also have considerable experience with the science that has evolved for defining the evidentiary basis for clinical practice. The attorneys are chosen because of a similar degree of accomplishment relating to the ethical, legal, and sociopolitical ramifications of medical decision making.

Membership in the CEP is a high honor, meant to be the highest honor that can be offered clinicians, since distinctions such as the Lasker or Nobel prizes do not target the clinical arena. It is also well compensated. These individuals bring extraordinary experiences, skills, and ethical probity to the task of rendering clinical decisions at a fiduciary level in real time. They have no fallback except to declare that they will revisit a particular decision sooner rather than later.

The CEP is designed to house the intellectual elite who can define the state of the science and the art of medicine and overlay a considerable patina of wisdom on behalf of individuals seeking care for covered illnesses. Determinations published by the CEP provide guidance to those who are administering the indemnity scheme and, even more important, provide information of substance to inform the doctor-patient dialogue regarding clinical decisions. The CEP is not tasked to approach any issues that relate to an individual patient.

The term of service for members of the CEP is five years without renewal. As retirement from the CEP approaches, the member will be expected to submit three names of candidates for replacement. Appointment follows a vote by the entire CEP and must be approved by the Workers' Compensation Commission. The CEP reports to the Workers' Compensation Commission and, pari-passu, to the executive branch housing the commission.

Efficacy Reviews

The CEP is responsive to inquiries as to the appropriateness of particular medical and surgical interventions submitted by the surgeon general, the Workers' Compensation Commission, or any of the members of the CEP itself. Each inquiry will be assigned to three members of the CEP: a pair of the medical professionals on the panel (one designated the primary and the other the secondary respondent) and a legal professional.

The primary reviewer is expected to extract relevant information from extant exercises in the Evidentiary Basis of Medical Practice, such as those catalogued by the Cochrane Collaboration and the ACP Journal Club. These might be supplemented by systematic studies published more recently than the available collections and analyses. It is not necessary nor expected that the reviewers undertake to reanalyze individual contributions to the relevant literature. They are tasked to explore this literature with the critical eye it deserves. Furthermore, that critical eye is conceptually driven, not analytically driven. It is not intended that they undertake systematic reviews of the systematic reviews, or meta-analyses of the meta-analyses. They are to delineate the limits of certainty regarding the efficacy of a particular intervention in a particular clinical setting.

The primary reviewer will summarize this information in a document to be reviewed by the secondary reviewer. Together, they will agree on the content of the document and express their opinion(s) as to the degree of efficacy. The legal professional will have access to the written interactions between the primary and secondary reviewers and be expected to contribute insights and guidance regarding validity, propriety, veracity, and substantiality. The resulting document is termed the Efficacy Review. The Efficacy Review will be distributed to all members of the CEP for perusal. All the deliberations entailed in producing these Efficacy Reviews will be considered privileged, since they may entail discussions that pertain to patient information.

Each medical member will serve as a primary respondent on three inquiries per month, ten months each year. Hence, an average of eighteen Efficacy Reviews will be produced each month. These will be distributed to all members of the CEP for review. The Efficacy Reviews will conclude with one of the following summary evaluations:

A. There is sound and substantial scientific (systematic) evidence suggesting a meaningful likelihood of clinically meaningful benefit.

B. There is substantial scientific evidence suggesting a statistically significant likelihood of benefit, but either the likelihood or the degree of benefit is marginal.

C. There is substantial scientific evidence suggesting that the intervention is ineffective and/or harmful.
D. There is no scientific support for efficacy, yet the intervention is common practice.
E. There is no scientific support for efficacy because the intervention is experimental. This would encompass many new devices and procedures that have not been subjected to scientific study, as well as interventions that are still actively under study.

It should be appreciated that all pharmaceutical interventions licensed by the FDA would qualify for a summary evaluation of "B"; some would be supported by sufficiently robust science to warrant an "A." The basis for licensing of devices by the FDA is less stringent, so the assumption of "B" does not operate.

Effectiveness Determinations

The Efficacy Reviews are an attempt to provide an estimation of the limitations of the relevant clinical science. This is a demanding exercise, particularly since the estimates of treatment outcomes are dependent on the analytic strategy underpinning the individual systematic review or meta-analysis.[7] In practice, the exercises that result in a summary evaluation grade of A, C, D, and E are relatively straightforward and noncontentious. However, most interventions that have been studied are graded B. And most interventions are studied in very defined and selected populations, selected often as to age, gender, presence of complicating conditions, and more. The usual practice in evidence-based medicine is to declare the science inadequate for a definitive recommendation as to appropriateness in clinical practice and to call for additional studies.

However, the CEP is mandated to make a definitive recommendation that will determine whether a UWCI carrier will allow or disallow coverage of the particular intervention. This is a determination that starts with the Efficacy Report, taking into account the quality of the evidence, estimates of the magnitude of beneficial and harmful effects in various populations, and the degree to which one has confidence in these estimates.[8] But the definitive recommendation demands more than the Efficacy Review can provide. It demands the application of judgment and wisdom, coupled with a fine moral compass. After all, the Efficacy Review is the result of judgments regarding the magnitude of particular clinical effects. Now we are superimposing an estimate of the value of these clinical effects to injured workers. Furthermore, the CEP operates under the fiduciary constraints of the UWCA. Is the intervention sufficiently efficacious that expenditure from the workers' aggregate and finite premium pool makes sense?

This question does not call for an actuarial or administrative answer. It is a question in the humanist tradition. It is a question laden with as many issues in moral relativism as in scientific validity. It speaks to the common good and demands a response in that context. This is the rationale for constituting the CEP, similar to the rational for supreme courts. These nine individuals must orchestrate a meeting of their minds that results in a definitive statement as to whether they feel the intervention is effective or ineffective.

To that end, the efficacy reviews are distributed to all members of the CEP. For two days each of ten months, the CEP will convene for a working session hosted by the Workers' Compensation Commission. The format for the meeting has the primary reviewer of each Efficacy Report, with contributions from the secondary and legal reviewers, presenting their assessment to the entire CEP for feedback. Each primary respondent will have two hours to present three reports. In the following month, the primary reviewer will revise the report accordingly and submit the revision to all members of the CEP for signature, now referred to as the Final Determination. The Final Determination shall be submitted to the commission for certification and publication.

The final determination will contain a Plain Language Summary designed to facilitate informed medical decision making on the part of the patient and the physician confronting the particular therapeutic option. The legal consultant who has overseen the particular Efficacy/ Final Report will serve the same role for the Plain Language Summary. After all, this is a document that will need to be readily comprehensible to many with interests vested in the particular intervention. The body of the Plain Language Summary is an evidence-based risk communication.[9]

The Plain Language Summary will include one of the following clinical recommendations:

1. This intervention has robust scientific support and should be offered and encouraged when clinically indicated. The treatment is effective.
2. This intervention has scientific support, but the support is either for infrequent benefit or benefit that is less than compelling. The recommendation as to whether a particular intervention in this category is deemed effective or ineffective is based on the frequency and magnitude of efficacy.
3. This intervention has been studied and, despite a degree of general acceptance, no clinically meaningful efficacy has been demonstrable. This intervention is ineffective.
4. This intervention has been subjected to comprehensive scientific studies. It appears that the clinical risks outweigh the clinical benefits. This intervention is ineffective.

If it is ineffective or harmful, it is not covered by UWCI. The worker may choose to seek coverage on a supplemental policy, a "wrap" purchased with their share of unexpended monies. But that is the worker's decision and money; it is not a shared expense.

Fee for Serving

The Final Determination is intended for purposes beyond arming the UWCI carrier, the Workers' Compensation Commission, and the state with guidance when designing coverage. It also serves to inform the physicians who have been enrolled to serve the medical needs of workers indemnified under UWCI and their patients who are indemnified by UWCI. Both will have access to all these documents whenever the need arises. It is likely that the UWCI carriers will provide an educational program that explains the approach and the fashion in which Final Determinations by the CEP inform clinical decisions. Aside from those interventions that are harmful, nothing is categorically excluded. The decision is to whether an intervention is covered by UWCI and, if covered, with what level of enthusiasm. Interventions that are deemed highly salutary are fully covered at rates similar to Medicare rates. Furthermore, the treating physician is not only paid automatically, just by entering personal identifying numbers into the UWCI website, but he or she also receives a bonus for practices that are well supported by evidence. The bonus is paid out piecemeal over time, but the fee for the encounter is paid instantly and without coding or other promoters of overhead expense. The UWCI considers the detection of inappropriate billing a far less important issue than appropriate care. Hence, if the prescribing physician ignores the inferences emanating from the CEP and prescribes less-efficacious options, there is no bonus. Of course, if the prescription is for the ineffective or the harmful, there is also no fee.

The intent is to create an environment that encourages productive, informed, and salutary relationships between physicians who are rewarded for ethical behavior and for active concern alongside patients, who are active participants in all matters that relate to their health. Ideally, patients will captain their ships with the physician as their navigator. Hubris and profit are to be defunded as much as possible.

This credo should rapidly capture the office practice of medicine. The inpatient experience is far too entrenched and ethically distorted to change readily. However, ethical office practice is the gatekeeper for most inpatient practices. When recourse to inpatient care is deemed advisable by the patient and physician, it should be provided regardless of the nonsense of coding, length-of-stay restrictions, and all else that has made the American hospital a business rather than a humanistic salve.

Planting the Flag of Medical Professionalism

UWCI is the best hope I can see for establishing a precedent for rational, compassionate health care. If it is successful, it will be because it inculcates precepts that were among the most worthy aspects of the iterations of the doctor-patient relationship we have visited in this book: "The Morning Prayer of the Physician," the traditions of humanism espoused in the introduction, the substantive science that was still a dream fifty years ago, and the reelevation of the patient-physician relationship to the moral high ground. "Health care" is neither an institution nor an industry. It is an accumulation of individual, always somewhat idiosyncratic, clinical events. Health care does not need to be institutionalized or industrialized. It should not succumb to profiteering or become predatory. Health care needs to be supported by an infrastructure that facilitates the doctor-patient dialogue and supports rational decisions that result. This is not a "service industry"; this is an enlightened monetization of altruism.

So, too, is the role of physician in the twenty-first century. It is time to cast off the "fee-for-service" rationalization and embrace fees for serving. If that happened, intangibles such as judgment, experience, and wisdom would be valued to the degree they deserve to be, and judged as only they can be judged: by peer review. Learning technical skills is far less difficult than learning when their application is appropriate. Instead of rewarding peers for the "doing," which predisposes to the doing, we must reward the quality of the consideration of the doing. This recruits the science of risks and benefits along with the ability to hear the values of a particular patient. That cognitive demand is common to all aspects of bedside medicine. That cognitive demand is the essence of fees for serving. It is why appointment to the CEP is such a high honor.

Enlightenment at the End
of the Tunnel
Guideposts for Future Physicians

I want to end this volume by offering my advice to the generations who will follow mine to the bedside of the patient. Composing another "Morning Prayer of the Physician" is anachronistic for the twenty-first century. Likewise, emulating the prose of a Martin Buber would strike too many involved in contemporary health care as inconsequential next to a Final Determination from a CEP. Even David Seegal's cartoons (figure 1) have grown more cute than weighty.

As I mentioned in chapter 6, about twenty years ago, I published "Four Laws of Therapeutic Dynamics." I've collected many more than four over the years. And today, rather than call them laws, I like to think of them as "guideposts for the perplexed physician." Here are some I cherish most:

Guidepost 1: Curb your dogma

This is not just about the contributions of scientific evidence to clinical practice. There's also concrete symbolism. The term "curbside consult" had been clinical vernacular for generations. The idea is that we should informally buttonhole a respected colleague when we have a clinical challenge. The curbside is the antidote for the malignant granularity of EPIC, the antithesis of dispassionate information technology. Any attempt to digitize the clinical record that denigrates the humanity of the clinical narrative is iatrogenic. The main reason for the clinical record is to remind you or a colleague, in the middle of the night or in six months, what you were thinking about and concerned about for the sake of your patient. Any other role for the digitized record is ancillary at best.

Curbside dialogue is the essence of professionalism and the only valid form of Continuing Medical Education. Furthermore, the curbside is where you can also care about your colleague's well-being. It's where eye contact can reveal the pain of disaffection, substance abuse, even suicidal ideation. Ours is a stressful mission, and beneath the white coat beats a very human heart. For us, collegiality has a therapeutic dimension.

Guidepost 2: Health care is not an industry or even a system

No one who is ill wants to be considered a "unit of care," and no one who cares wants to be called a "provider." You may go to clinic, or the operating room, or the office, but you don't go to work. And you don't bring work home; the same critical and empathic mindset walks through the door at the end of the day as it did at the beginning. You are expected to participate in valuing options in complex situations at the bedside; you are fortunate to have such skills to bring home. If complexities are overwhelming, find the appropriate curbside.

Health care is an interactive community of unique professionals that exists for one purpose: to care for the unique individuals who present themselves for caring. That's why you went into medicine. Don't lose sight of that in the "six sigma" sophisms.

No physician should have "cases." No physician should treat "diseases." Physicians treat people who have chosen to be their patients. Objectifying their plight is necessary, but treating patients so they end up people again, even people with diseases, is the goal.

Guidepost 3: Health is not a diagnosis

Americans believe that they should be free of morbidity from birth until that fateful eighty-fifth birthday. Americans and their physicians need to be disabused of that fantasy. We now have a science that informs the definition of "health." One of the pioneering studies, the "Health in Detroit" study, was published nearly forty years ago by Lois Verbrugge and her colleagues in Ann Arbor. They asked some

600 people to keep a diary for six weeks in which, at bedtime, they recorded every miserable thing that happened to them that day. We now have a great deal of information of this nature. If anyone goes a year without a backache, it's abnormal. Three years without a month of knee or shoulder pain, that's abnormal. If you go a year without headache, heartache, heartburn, or something unpleasant with your bowels, that's abnormal. Health is not the avoidance of morbidity; health is having the wherewithal to cope with the next predicament and to cope so well that it is not long memorable.

That requires an inherent sense of invincibility. This sense of invincibility is far more fragile than organ-system homeostasis. This sense of invincibility has always been a target for medicalization, and never more so than today. Everyone is burdened by baggage garnered from the Internet, television, Oprah, Dr. Oz, and all the other New Age oracles who proclaim the scare of the week and the miracle of the month. You can't eat, drink, or breathe anything without considering its implications for your health. That's why so many are comfortable shopping in the placebo aisle at Whole Foods. This is a cacophony that challenges coping. The next predicament can seem to be the last straw, and recourse, even recourse to a physician, can become the only sensible option. If the decision is to go to a physician, the physician's mandate is to understand why the person has come. For example, when a person seeks medical care and announces "My back is killing me, Doc," could it be that the chief complaint actually is, "My back is killing me, Doc, and I can't cope with this episode"?

Guidepost 4: Fees for listening, then serving

No one chooses the role of patient for the fun of it. Short of catastrophe, a person allows herself to become a patient because she has failed to come up with a satisfying diagnosis and therapeutic plan on her own. Every symptom has been tempered by your patient's preconceptions and distorted by yours. If you are not prepared to listen, you will be misled by surrogate symptoms.

For example, consider grandma's knee pain. If you compare the knees of elderly women who choose to be patients with knee pain with the knees of elderly women with knee pain in the community who do not seek medical advice, there is no important anatomical difference. The difference between the elderly woman with knee pain who becomes a patient and the elderly woman who remains a person is often contextual; it reflects a compromise in coping ability. Perhaps there is unresolved grief or consternation when social or physical support has diminished. The arthroscope is not a reasonable solution. Isn't the arthroscopist more valuable for realizing that than for performing arthroscopy?

The twenty-first century can support a new doctor-patient relationship, one where the patient is captain of the ship and the doctor is the navigator. The patient should understand the limits of certainty regarding medical options and be in a position to value options personally. A trusting relationship between doctor and patient is always palliative. Don't ever imagine that your demeanor, eye contact, attentiveness, and persona are not essential to any treatment act. Usually, we call this bedside manner.

THERE ARE MORE GUIDEPOSTS I could discuss, and many more you will discover on your own. All you need is a commitment to caring about and for those in need. Life as a physician allows little room for self-indulgence. For those of you who are drawn to a career anchored at the bedside, the trade-off is the quiet, internalized quest to become a better physician.

I am a serious believer in your generation and what you will accomplish for patient care. No matter how exhausted or hurried you feel, take comfort in the privilege society has given you to be responsible for providing a fellow human being a port in a storm. Doing that well is its own reward. Doing that well carries over into every other aspect of your life.

NOTES

ABBREVIATIONS

Ann Intern Med	*Annals of Internal Medicine*
BMJ	*British Medical Journal*
JAMA	*Journal of the American Medical Association*
J Occup Environ Med	*Journal of Occupational and Environmental Medicine*
N Engl J Med	*New England Journal of Medicine*

INTRODUCTION

1. This is the title of the valedictory address delivered by Sir William Osler at the University of Pennsylvania's school of medicine on May 1, 1889. It is well worth reading today. It can be accessed from the medical archives of the Johns Hopkins Medical Institute (www.medicalarchives.jhmi.edu/osler/aequessay.htm). We will return to this essay later in the chapter.

2. A. N. Whitehead, *Science and the Modern World* (1925; New York: Free Press, 1997).

3. N. Tomes, "Patient Empowerment and the Dilemmas of Late-Modern Medicalization," *The Lancet* 369 (2007): 698–700.

4. M. Lipkin, *The Care of Patients: Perspectives and Practices* (New Haven: Yale University Press, 1987).

5. L. Thomas, *The Youngest Science: Notes of a Medicine-Watcher* (New York: Viking Press, 1983).

6. E. H. Erikson, "The Nature of Clinical Evidence," *Daedalus* 87 (1958): 65–87

CHAPTER 1

1. Annual American Hospital Association Survey of Hospitals, "Hospitals and Other Health Facilities," *Medical Care Research and Review* 17 (1960): 463–71.

2. R. Porter, "Major Revision in Hospital Use Sought for New York City," *New York Times*, August 5, 1960.

3. P. E. Dans, "David Seegal. Ic ne wat and Other Maxims of a Master Teacher," *The Pharos* (Autumn 2014): 4–8.

4. C. Gray, "Streetscapes: Morrisania Hospital; A Tidy Relic of the 1920's Looking for a New Use," *New York Times*, July 15, 1990.

5. C. E. Rosenberg, *The Care of Strangers: The Rise of America's Hospital System* (New York: Basic Books, 1987).

6. V. Rodwin, *Public Hospital Systems in New York and Paris* (New York: New York University Press, 1992).

7. M. Balint, "The Doctor, His Patient, and the Illness," *The Lancet* (April 2, 1955): 683–88.

8. A. Kleinman, "Medicine's Symbolic Reality: A Central Problem in the Philosophy of Medicine," *Inquire* 16 (1973): 206–13; A. Kleinman, *The Illness Narratives* (New York: Basic Books, 1988).

9. A. Kleinman, "From Illness as Culture to Caregiving as Moral Experience," *N Engl J Med* 368 (2013): 1376–77.

CHAPTER 2

1. N. M. Hadler, "Genetic Influence on Phototaxis in Drosophila Melanogaster," *Biological Bulletin* 126 (1964): 264–73; N. M. Hadler, "Heritability and Phototaxis in Drosophila Melanogaster," *Genetics* 50 (1964): 1269–77.

2. K. M. Ludmerer, *Learning to Heal: The Development of American Medical Education* (New York: Basic Books, 1985); K. M. Ludmerer, *Time to Heal: American Medical Education from the Turn of the Century to the Era of Managed Care* (Oxford, UK: Oxford University Press, 2005).

3. http://www.amednews.com/article/20091109/profession/311099981/5/.

4. http://www.thecrimson.com/article/1966/6/16/education-at-the-medical-school-pithis/.

5. I. J. Lewis and C. G. Sheps, *The Sick Citadel: The American Academic Medical Center and the Public Interest* (Cambridge, Mass.: Oelgeschlager Gunn & Hain, 1983).

6. N. M. Hadler, *The Citizen Patient: Reforming Health Care for the Sake of the Patient, Not the System* (Chapel Hill: University of North Carolina Press, 2013).

7. The "medical service" is the purview of the Department of Medicine and houses patients with diseases that are considered most appropriate for the ministrations of specialists in internal medicine and its subspecialties (rheumatology, cardiology, gastroenterology, endocrinology, infectious diseases, hematology, and oncology).

8. S. R. Moonesinghe, J. Lowery, N. Shahi, and others, "Impact of Reduction in Working Hours for Doctors in Training on Postgraduate Medical Education and Patients' Outcomes: Systematic Review," *BMJ* 342 (2011): d1580 (doi:10.1136/bmj.d1580).

9. L. Axelrod, D. J. Shah, and A. B Jena, "The European Working Time Directive: An Uncontrolled Experiment in Medical Care and Education," *JAMA* 309 (2013): 447–48.

CHAPTER 3

1. N. M. Hadler, *The Citizen Patient: Reforming Health Care for the Sake of the Patient, Not the System* (Chapel Hill: University of North Carolina Press, 2013).

2. D. S. Jones, *Broken Hearts: The Tangled History of Cardiac Care* (Baltimore: Johns Hopkins University Press, 2013).

3. http://thehealthcareblog.com/blog/2013/10/13/the-end-of-the-coronary-angi
oplasty-era/; http://thehealthcareblog.com/blog/2013/10/19/the-great-coronary-an
gioplasty-debate-giving-patients-the-right-to-choose/.

4. N. M. Hadler, "De Morte Medicine," *Clinical Research* 32 (1984): 9–12.

5. N. M. Hadler, "The Extinction of the Physician," *North Carolina Medical Journal* 45 (1984): 124–25.

6. http://www.amednews.com/article/20080107/profession/301079974/5/; http://
www.amednews.com/article/20091109/profession/311099981/5/.

7. L. Payer, *Medicine and Culture* (New York: Henry Holt, 1988).

8. N. M. Hadler, "Reflections of an American Educator at the Japanese Bedside,"
The Pharos 57 (1994): 9–13.

CHAPTER 4

1. N. M. Hadler, "Medicine's Industrial Revolution Is Here: Rally the Luddites,"
J Occup Environ Med 36 (1994): 1038–40.

2. N. M. Hadler, *Occupational Musculoskeletal Disorders*, 3rd ed. (Philadelphia:
Lippincott, Williams & Wilkins, 2005); N. M. Hadler, *Stabbed in the Back: Confront-
ing Back Pain in an Overtreated Society* (Chapel Hill: University of North Carolina
Press, 2009).

3. E. C. Rich, M. Liebow, M. Srinivasan, and others, "Medicare Financing of Graduate Medical Education," *Journal of General Internal Medicine* 17 (2002): 283–92.

4. P. J. Perry and C. A. Wilborn, "Sorotonin Syndrome vs. Neuroleptic Malignant
Syndrome: A Contrast of Causes, Diagnoses, and Management," *Annals of Clinical
Psychiatry* 24 (2012): 155–62.

5. D. A. Asch and R. M. Parker, "The Libby Zion Case: One Step Forward or Two
Steps Backward?," *N Engl J Med* 318 (1988): 771–75.

6. L. Rosenbaum and D. Lamas, "Residents' Duty Hours—Toward an Empirical
Narrative," *N Engl J Med* 367 (2012): 2044–49.

7. L. Axelrod, D. J. Shah, and A. B. Jena, "The European Working Time Directive: An
Uncontrolled Experiment in Medical Care and Education," *JAMA* 309 (2013): 447–48.

8. http://www.rcseng.ac.uk/news/impact-of-doctor-working-time-cap-on-patient-
safety-and-training-getting-worse-says-new-survey (accessed February 20, 2014).

9. L. I. Horwitz, "Does Improving Handoffs Reduce Medical Error Rates?," *JAMA*
310 (2013): 2255–56.

10. A. J. Starmer, T. C. Sectish, D. W. Simon, and others, "Rates of Medical Errors
and Preventable Adverse Events among Hospitalized Children following the Implementation of a Resident Handoff Bundle," *JAMA* 310 (2013): 2262–70; G. Dhaliwal
and K. E. Hauer, "The Oral Patient Presentation in the Era of Night Float Admissions," *JAMA* 310 (2013): 2247–48.

11. R. Wachter and L. Goldman, "The Emerging Role of 'Hospitalists' in the
American Health Care System," *N Engl J Med* 335 (1996): 514–17.

12. M. S. Patel, K. G. Volpp, D. S. Small, and others, "Association of the 2011
ACGME Resident Duty Hour Reforms with Mortality and Readmissions among

Hospitalized Medicare Patients," *JAMA* 312 (2014): 2364–73; R. Rajaram, J. W. Chung, A. T. Jones, and others, "Association of the 2011 ACGME Resident Duty Hour Reforms with General Surgery Patient Outcomes and with Resident Examination Performance," *JAMA* 312 (2014): 2374–84.

13. S. V. Desai, L. Feldma, L. Brown, and others, "Effect of the 2011 vs. 2003 Duty Hour Regulation-Compliant Models on Sleep Duration, Trainee Education, and Continuity of Patient Care among Internal Medicine House Staff: A Randomized Trial," *JAMA Internal Medicine* 173 (2013): 649–55.

14. B. C. Drolet, M. T. Khokhar, and S. A. Fischer, "The 2011 Duty-Hour Requirements—A Survey of Residency Program Directors," *N Engl J Med* 368 (2013): 694–97.

15. V. Johnson, "A Resitern's Reflections on Duty-Hours Reform," *N Engl J Med* 369 (2013): 2278–79.

16. V. M. Arora, J. M. Farnan, and H. F. Humphrey, "Professionalism in the Era of Duty Hours: Time for a Shift Change?," *JAMA* 308 (2012): 2195–96; P. Klass, "Getting through the Night," *N Engl J Med* 369 (2013): 2279–80.

17. N. A. Buckley, A. Dawson, and G. K. Isbister, "Serotonin Syndrome," *BMJ* 348 (2014): g1626 (doi:10.1136/bmj.g1626).

18. National Research Council, *To Err Is Human: Building a Safer Health System* (Washington, D.C.: National Academies Press, 2000).

19. National Research Council, *Crossing the Quality Chasm: A New Health System for the 21st Century* (Washington, D.C: National Academies Press, 2001).

20. https://oig.hhs.gov/oei/reports/oei-06-09-00090.pdf.

21. J. T. James, "A New, Evidence-Based Estimate of Patient Harms Associated with Hospital Care," *Journal of Patient Safety* 9 (2013): 122–28 (doi:10.1097/PTS.0b013e3182948a69).

22. Y. Wang, N. Eldridge, M. L. Metersky, and others, "National Trends in Patient Safety for Four Common Conditions, 2005–2011," *N Engl J Med* 370 (2014): 341–51.

23. D. R. Urbach, A. Govindarajan, R. Saskin, A. S. Wilton, and N. N. Baxter, "Introduction of Surgical Safety Checklists in Ontario, Canada," *N Engl J Med* 370 (2014): 1029–38.

24. L. Leape, "The Checklist Conundrum," *N Engl J Med* 370 (2014): 1063–64.

25. R. A. Hayward and T. P. Hofer, "Estimating Hospital Deaths due to Medical Errors," *JAMA* 286 (2001): 415–20.

26. R. A. Gooch and J. M. Kahn, "ICU Bed Supply, Utilization, and Health Care Spending: An Example of Demand Elasticity," *JAMA* 311 (2014): 567–68.

CHAPTER 5

1. J. B. Colla, A. C. Bracken, L. M. Kinney, and W. B. Weeks, "Measuring Patient Safety Climate: A Review of Surveys," *Quality and Safety in Health Care* 14 (2005): 364–66.

2. D. C. Classen, R. Resar, F. Griffin, and others, "'Global Trigger Tool' Shows That Adverse Events in Hospitals May Be Ten Times Greater than Previously Measured," *Health Affairs* 30 (2011): 581–89.

3. http://asqhdandl.org/uploads/3/3/3/8/3338526/leadership_and_profound_knowledge_final_b_opt.pdf.

4. C. D. DeAngelis, "Conflicts of Interest in Medical Practice and Their Costs to the Nation's Health and Health Care System," *Milbank Quarterly* 92 (2014): 195–98.

5. See L. Rosenbaum, "Reconnecting the Dots—Reinterpreting Industry-Physician Relations," *N Engl J Med* 372 (2015): 1860–64; "Understanding Bias—The Case for Careful Study," *N Engl J Med* 372 (2015): 1959–63; and "Beyond Moral Outrage—Weighing the Trade-Offs of COI Regulation," *N Engl J Med* 372 (2015): 2064–68.

6. http://thehealthcareblog.com/blog/2013/10/13/the-end-of-the-coronary-angioplasty-era/.

7. http://blogs.scientificamerican.com/guest-blog/2013/11/22/how-clinical-guidelines-can-fail-both-doctors-and-patients/.

8. E. D. Pisano, R. N. Golden, and L. Schweitzer, "Conflict of Interest Policies for Academic Health System Leaders Who Work with Outside Corporations," *JAMA* 311 (2014): 1111–12.

9. D. Armstrong, "PepsiCo Director Quitting to Lead Health Institute That Touted Soda Tax," *Bloomberg Businessweek*, February 21, 2014.

10. E. G. Campbell, J. S. Weissman, S. Ehringhaus, S. R. Rao, B. Moy, S. Feibelmann, and S. D. Goold, "Institutional Academic Industry Relationships," *JAMA* 298 (2007): 1779–86.

11. D. Korn and D. Carlat, "Conflicts of Interest in Medical Education: Recommendations from the Pew Task Force on Medical Conflicts of Interest," *JAMA* 310 (2013): 2397–98.

CHAPTER 6

1. P. A. Cohen, "Hazards of Hindsight—Monitoring the Safety of Nutritional Supplements," *N Engl J Med* 370 (2014): 1277–80.

2. American Association of Medical Colleges, "The State of Health Equity Research: Closing Knowledge Gaps to Address Inequities" (American Association of Medical Colleges [www.aamc.org], 2014), 1–15.

3. R. Wilkinson and K. Pickett, *The Spirit Level: Why Equality Is Better for Everyone* (London: Bloomsbury Press, 2011); N. Krieger, *Epidemiology and the People's Health* (New York: Oxford University Press, 2011).

4. N. M. Hadler, "Benefits That Do Not Benefit," *J Occup Environ Med* 56 (2014): e16–17.

5. N. M. Hadler, "Four Laws of Therapeutic Dynamics," *J Occup Environ Med* 39 (1997): 295–98.

6. http://www.mckinsey.com/insights/business_technology/big_data_the_next_frontier_for_innovation.

7. http://www.mckinsey.com/insights/health_systems_and_services/accounting_for_the_cost_of_us_health_care.

8. E. C. Stecker and S. A. Schroeder, "Adding Value to Relative-Value Units," *N Engl J Med* 369 (2013): 2176–78.

9. M. B. Rothberg, P. S. Pekow, A. Priya, and P. K. Lindenauer, "Variation in Diagnostic Coding of Patients with Pneumonia and Its Association with Hospital Risk-Standardized Mortality Rates," *Ann Intern Med* 160 (2014): 380–88.

10. R. Kaushal, "Reducing the Costs of U.S. Health Care: The Role of Electronic Health Records," *Ann Intern Med* 159 (2013): 151–52.

11. R. Koppel, "Demanding Utility from Health Information Technology," *Ann Intern Med* 158 (2013): 845–46.

12. J. Adler-Milstein, C. Salzber, C. Granz, E. J. Orav, J. P. Newhouse, and D. W. Bates, "Effect of Electronic Health Records on Health Care Costs: Longitudinal Comparative Evidence from Community Practice," *Ann Intern Med* 159 (2013): 97–104.

13. A. L. Kellermann and S. S. Jones, "What It Will Take to Achieve As-Yet-Unfulfilled Promises of Health Information Technology," *Health Affairs* 32 (2013): 63–68.

14. R. Hillesta, J. Bigelow, A. Bower, F. Girosi, R. Meil, R. Scoville, and others, "Can Electronic Medical Record Systems Transform Health Care? Potential Health Benefits, Savings, and Costs," *Health Affairs* 24 (2005): 1103–17.

15. J. A. Linder, J. Ma, D. W. Bates, B. Middleton, and R. S. Stafford, "Electronic Health Record Use and the Quality of Ambulatory Care in the United States," *Archives of Internal Medicine* 167 (2007): 1400–1405; R. D. Cebul, T. E. Love, A. K. Jain, and C. J. Hebert, "Electronic Health Records and Quality of Diabetes Care," *N Engl J Med* 365 (2011): 825–33.

16. S. S. Jones, R. S. Rudin, T. Perry, and P. G. Shekelle, "Health Information Technology: An Updated Systematic Review with a Focus on Meaningful Use," *Ann Intern Med* 160 (2014): 48–54.

17. M. H. Beckmann, J. J. Westbrook, Y. Koh, C. Lo, and R. O. Day, "Does Computerized Provider Order Entry Reduce Prescribing Errors for Hospital Inpatients? A Systematic Review," *Journal of the American Medical Informatics Association* 16 (2009): 613–23.

18. J. Millman and D. S. Fallis, "Doctors React to Release of Medicare Billing Records," *Washington Post*, April 9, 2014.

CHAPTER 7

1. Joe Selby, *PCORI's Research Will Answer Patients' Real-World Questions* (Health Affairs Blog, March 29, 2014; copyright © 2014 Health Affairs by Project HOPE—The People-to-People Health Foundation, Inc.).

2. http://thehealthcareblog.com/blog/2010/01/11/comparative-effectiveness-research-and-kindred-delusions/#more.

3. Z. Moukheiber, "EPIC System's Tough Billionaire," *Forbes Magazine*, http://www.forbes.com/sites/zinamoukheiber/2012/04/18/epic-systems-tough-billionaire/.

4. http://thehealthcareblog.com/blog/2013/10/13/the-end-of-the-coronary-angioplasty-era/; http://thehealthcareblog.com/blog/2013/10/19/the-great-coronary-angioplasty-debate-giving-patients-the-right-to-choose/.

5. http://blogs.scientificamerican.com/guest-blog/2013/11/22/how-clinical-guidelines-can-fail-both-doctors-and-patients/.

6. http://www.iom.edu/Reports/2011/Clinical-Practice-Guidelines-We-Can-Trust/Standards.aspx.

7. P. S. Roshanov, N. Fernandes, J. M. Wilczynski, B. J. Hemens, and others, "Features of Effective Computerized Clinical Decision Support Systems: Meta-Regression of 162 Randomised Trials," *BMJ* 346 (2013): 1657–69.

8. S. J. Katz, "Treatment Decision Aids Are Unlikely to Cut Healthcare Costs: We Should Be Asking Broader Questions about Quality and Effectiveness," *BMJ* 348 (2014): g1172/bmj.g1172.

9. P. Croskerry, "From Mindless to Mindful Practice—Cognitive Bias and Clinical Decision Making," *N Engl J Med* 368 (2013): 2445–48.

10. S. B. Abramson, D. Jacob, M. Rosenfeld, and others, "A 3-year M.D.—Accelerating Careers, Diminishing Debt," *N Engl J Med* 369 (2013): 1085–87; J. Hamblin, "Dr. Howser's Army: The 3-Year M.D.," *Atlantic*, September 30, 2013.

11. R. B. Doherty and R. A. Crowley for the Health and Public Policy Committee of the American College of Physicians, "Principles Supporting Dynamic Clinical Care Teams: An American College of Physicians Position Paper," *Ann Intern Med* 159 (2013): 620–26; A. Reisman, "Championing Truly Collaborative Team-Based Care," *Ann Intern Med* 159 (2013): 642–43.

12. M. Smith, G. Halvorson, and G. Kaplan, "What's Needed Is a Health Care System That Learns," *JAMA* 308 (2012): 1637–38.

13. D. Korn and D. Carlat, "Conflicts of Interest in Medical Education: Recommendations from the Pew Task Force on Medical Conflicts of Interest," *JAMA* 310 (2013): 2397–98.

14. D. A. Asch and D. F. Weinstein, "Innovation in Medical Education," *N Engl J Med* 371 (2014): 794–95.

15. N. M. Pageler, C. P. Friedman, and C. A. Longhurst, "Refocusing Medical Education in the EMR Era," *JAMA* 310 (2013): 2249–50.

16. www.abim.org/program-directors-administrators/milestones.aspx.

17. K. J. Caverzagie, W. F. Lobst, E. M. Aagaard, and others, "The Internal Medicine Reporting Milestones and the Next Accreditation System," *Ann Intern Med* 158 (2013): 557–59.

18. C. D. DeAngelis, "The Electronic Health Record: Boom or Bust for Good Patient Care?," *Milbank Quarterly* 92 (2014): 442–45.

19. B. M. Gray, J. L. Vandergrift, M. M. Johnston, and others, "Association between Imposition of Maintenance of Certification Requirement and Ambulatory Care-Sensitive Hospitalizations and Health Care Costs," *JAMA* 312 (2014): 2348–57; J. Hayes, J. L. Jackson, G. M. McNutt, and others, "Association between Physician Time-Unlimited vs. Time-Limited Internal Medicine Board Certification and Ambulatory Patient Care Quality," *JAMA* 312 (2014): 2358–63.

CHAPTER 8

1. http://blogs.scientificamerican.com/guest-blog/2013/05/29/the-scientific-basis-for-choosing-to-be-a-patient-forearmed-is-forewarned/.

2. A. Gelman and E. Loken, "The Statistical Crisis in Science," *American Scientist* 102 (2014): 460–65.

3. E. Y. Adashi and R. P. Kocher, "Physician Self-Referral: Regulation by Exceptions," *JAMA* (published online, January 12, 2015; doi:10.1001/jama.2014.16600).

4. F. Mostashari, D. Sanghavi, and M. McClellan, "Health Reform and Physician-Led Accountable Care," *JAMA* 311 (2014): 1855–56.

5. M. DeCamp, J. Sugarman, and S. Berkowitz, "Shared Savings in Accountable Care Organizations," *JAMA* 311 (2014): 1011–12.

6. M. Roland and S. Campbell, "Successes and Failures of Par for Performance in the United Kingdom," *N Engl J Med* 370 (2014): 1944–49.

7. D. Loxterkamp, "Humanism in the Time of Metrics," *BMJ* 347 (2013): 15539 (doi:10.1136/bmj.15539).

8. M. W. Friedberg, E. C. Schneider, M. B. Rosenthal, K. G. Volpp, and R. M. Werner, "Association between Participation in a Multipayer Medical Home Intervention and Changes in Quality, Utilization, and Costs of Care," *JAMA* 311 (2014): 815–25.

9. T. L. Schwenk, "The Patient-Centered Medical Home: One Size Does Not Fit All," *JAMA* 311 (2014): 802–3.

10. R. J. Baron and K. Davis, "Accelerating the Adoption of High Value Primary Care—A New Provider Type under Medicare?," *N Engl J Med* 370 (2014): 99–101.

11. A. Kleinman, "From Illness as Culture to Caregiving as Moral Experience," *N Engl J Med* 368 (2013): 1376–77.

12. http://www.nybooks.com/articles/archives/2014/feb/06/on-breaking-ones-neck/.

13. N. Biller-Andorno and T. H. Lee, "Ethical Physician Incentives—From Carrots and Sticks to Shared Purpose," *N Engl J Med* 368 (2013): 980–82.

CHAPTER 9

1. N. M. Hadler, "The Health Assurance, Disease Insurance Plan: Harnessing Reason to the Benefits of Employees," *J Occup Environ Med* 47 (2005): 655–57.

2. http://www.nap.edu/openbook.php?record_id=13444&page=102.

3. A. R. Feinstein, *Clinimetrics* (New Haven: Yale University Press, 1987).

4. N. M. Hadler, "Health Assurance and the Communitarian Ethic," *J Occup Environ Med* 50 (2008): 1096–98.

5. N. M. Hadler, *Occupational Musculoskeletal Disorders*, 3rd ed. (Philadelphia: Lippincott and Wilkins, 2005); N. M. Hadler, *Stabbed in the Back: Confronting Back Pain in an Overtreated Society* (Chapel Hill: University of North Carolina Press, 2009).

6. L. C. Baker and A. B. Kreuger, "Twenty-Four Hour Coverage and Workers' Compensation Insurance," *Health Affairs* 12 (1993): 271–81; D. T. Ballen, "Sleeper Issue in Health Care Reform: The Threat to Workers' Compensation," *Cornell Law Review* 79 (1994): 1291–1302.

7. J. A. Berlin and R. M. Golub, "Meta-Analysis as Evidence: Building a Better Pyramid," *JAMA* 312 (2014): 603–4; A. Deschartres, D. G. Altman, L. Trinquart,

I. Boutron, and P. Ravaud, "Association between Analytic Strategy and Estimates of Treatment Outcomes in Meta-Analyses," *JAMA* 312 (2014): 623–30.

8. M. H. Murad, V. M. Montori, J. P. A. Ioannidis, and others, "How to Read a Systematic Review and Meta-Analysis and Apply the Results to Patient Care," *JAMA* 312 (2014): 171–79.

9. D. A. Zipkin, C. A. Unscheid, N. L. Keating, and others, "Evidence-Based Risk Communication: A Systematic Review," *Ann Intern Med* 161 (2014): 270–80.

ABOUT THE AUTHOR

Nortin M. Hadler, M.D., M.A.C.P., M.A.C.R., F.A.C.O.E.M., is a graduate of Yale College and the Harvard Medical School. He trained at the Massachusetts General Hospital, the National Institutes of Health, and the Clinical Research Centre in London. He was certified a Diplomate of the American Boards of Internal Medicine, Rheumatology, Allergy & Immunology and Geriatrics. He joined the faculty of the University of North Carolina in 1973 and was promoted to professor of medicine and microbiology/immunology in 1985. He transitioned to emeritus status in 2015. During his career at UNC, he served as attending rheumatologist at the University of North Carolina Hospitals. Teaching at the bedside to all levels of students of medicine has been a focus of his professional life, recognized by multiple awards for these activities at UNC and elsewhere. In recognition of his clinical activities, he was elevated to Mastership in both the American College of Physicians and the American College of Rheumatology.

The molecular biology of hyaluran and the immunobiology of peptidoglycans were the focus of Dr. Hadler's early investigative career. Because of the contributions of his laboratory, he was selected as an established investigator of the American Heart Association and elected to membership in the American Society for Clinical Investigation. The focus on basic biology was superseded by what he initially termed "industrial rheumatology." Over 200 papers and twelve books bear witness to his analyses of "the illness of work incapacity," including the sociopolitical constraints imposed by various nations faced with the challenges of applying disability and compensation insurance schemes to predicaments such as back pain and arm pain in the workplace, as well as for a more global illness narrative such as is labeled "fibromyalgia." Dr. Hadler is widely regarded for his critical assessment of the limitations of certainty regarding medical and surgical management of the regional musculoskeletal disorders. The third edition of his monograph *Occupational Musculoskeletal Disorders* was published by Lippincott Williams & Wilkins in 2005 and provides a ready resource as to his thinking on the regional musculoskeletal disorders. In recognition of this work, he was elected to the National Academy of Social Insurance and is a fellow of the American College of Occupational and Environmental Medicine.

Dr. Hadler has lectured widely, including many named lectureships, and is a frequent commentator for the print and broadcast media. He has garnered multiple awards and served lengthy visiting professorships in England, France, Israel, and Japan.

Fifteen years ago, he turned his critical razor to much that is considered contemporary medicine at its finest. Assaults on medicalization and overtreatment have appeared in many editorials and commentaries and in five monographs: McGill-Queens University Press published *The Last Well Person: How to Stay Well Despite the Health-Care System* in 2004 (paperback, 2007). UNC Press published *Worried Sick: A Prescription for Health in an Overtreated America* (2008; paperback, 2012); *Stabbed in the Back: Confronting Back Pain in an Overtreated Society* (2009); *Rethinking Aging: Growing Old and Living Well in an Overtreated Society* (2011); and *Citizen Patient: Reforming Health Care for the Sake of the Patient, Not the System* (2013). Les Presses de l'Université Laval published the French translations of these works: *Le Dernier des bien portants* (2008), *Malades d'inquiétude* (2010), *Poignardé dans le dos* (2011; won Prix Prescrire in 2012), *Repenser le vieillissement* (2013), and *Citoyen et patient* (2014).

By the Bedside of the Patient is written at the request of readers of these books. Many are students and physicians in training who desired an understanding of how the social construction of "the doctor" has evolved, as seen through Dr. Hadler's eyes, decade by decade since the 1950s. As he points out, during those decades, health has become a commodity, disease a product line, and doctors a sales force. Dr. Hadler's earlier books take on the first two imprecations; *By the Bedside of the Patient* deals with the third.

The publication of *By the Bedside of the Patient* occurs in a watershed year in Dr. Hadler's career. In 2015 he assumed a leadership role in an initiative designed to provide rational health care in an evidence-based, cost-effective, employer-sponsored, defined-contribution, health-insurance scheme for the benefit of the patient. Chapter 9 of this book discusses the details and implications of such a model for patient-centered care.

INDEX

Italic page numbers indicate illustrations.

"Big Data: The Next Frontier for Innovation, Competition, and Productivity" (report), 114

Billing: digital, 120–27; in Universal Workers' Compensation Insurance, 174–75. *See also* Fee structures

Biostatistics, 104

Body Mass Index (BMI), 109

Bonuses, physician, in Universal Workers' Compensation Insurance, 174–75

Boston City Hospital (BCH), Harvard Service at, 12, 40–41

Boston Lying-in Hospital, 23

Boston Medical and Surgical Journal, 14

Bowdoin College, 22

Brandeis University, 20

British Medical Journal, 147–48

Bronx. *See* New York City

Buber, Martin, 157, 177

Bulfinch, Charles, 43

Bush, George H. W., 124

Business models, health-care: alternative proposals for, 152–55; consolidation in, 112–20; multispecialty and group practice, 150–52; private practice, 58, 117, 150–52

California, workers' compensation in, 166–67

Carder, Brooks, 95

Cardiology, interventional: marketing of, 137; rise of, 54–55, 70

"Care of the Patient, The" (Peabody), 12

Carnegie Foundation, 21

Carolinas Healthcare System, 119

Cassel, Christine, 97

Castle, William B., 40

Centers for Disease Control (CDC), 56–57

Centers for Medicare and Medicaid Services (CMS), 96, 99–100

CEP. *See* Clinical Effectiveness Panel

Cerner, 132

Certainty, limits of, 4, 6, 45, 169, 171, 180

Certification, maintenance of (MOC), 142–44

Charge nurses, 66, 68

Charity care, 44, 53, 55–56

Chauvinism, 73

Checklists, safety, 90–91

Chivian, Eric, 36

Clerkships, clinical, 34, 37–42

Cleveland Clinic, 55, 133

Clinic(s): freestanding, of specialists, 101, 151; patient-centered, 152. *See also* Private practice

Clinical competence: attempts to quantify, 140–44, *142, 143*; peer review of, 69, 140

Clinical education, 75–93; in 1960s, 34, 37–42; in 1970s and 1980s, 62–71; clinical investigation in, 47–48; in Japan, 71–74; limits on hours worked and, 45–46, 79–89; and medical errors, 89–92; Medicare's effects on, 55–56, 77–79; rise of assault on, 75–79; specialists in, 70–71. *See also* Teaching hospitals

Clinical Effectiveness Panel (CEP), 169–76

Clinical effectiveness research (CER), 130–32

Clinical Methods (Hutchison), 147

Clinical trials, 102–7; clinically meaningful benefits in, 104–7; conflicts of interest in, 105–7; FDA licensing and, 104–7, 129–30; recruitment of subjects for, 103; small effects in, 102–4; translational research in, 102–4, 107

Clinimetrics Units, 162–63, 169

CME. *See* Continuing Medical Education

Code of Medical Ethics, AMA, 53

Coding, medical, 121–24

Cohen, Julius, 20, 22–23, 29

Coler Hospital, 26
Columbia University, 24, 40–41
Commerce, Department of, 112
Commodification, of health, 3, 145
Competence. *See* Clinical competence
Computerized provider order entry
    (CPOE), 126, 138
Computers, in decision making, 135,
    138. *See also* Electronic records
Cone Health, 119
Conflicts of interest: in clinical trials,
    105–7; in Continuing Medical
    Education, 59–60; in digital
    invoicing, 124–25; in evaluation of
    quality of care, 96–99; in pharma-
    ceutical industry, 59, 101–2, 105–7;
    problems with admission of, 59–60
Congress: and attending physicians, 77;
    and medical errors, 89; and workers'
    compensation, 164. *See also specific
    laws*
Consulting firms, health-care manage-
    ment, 112–13, 114–15
Continuing Medical Education (CME):
    conflicts of interest in, 59–60;
    curbside consults as form of, 178;
    medical school education as
    foundation for, 35; quantifying
    competency in, 142–44; rise of, 59
Continuity of care, limits on physician
    hours and, 81–84
Contracted research organizations
    (CROs), 103, 105–6
Co-pays, 126, 168
Coping, with illness, 178–80
Cornell Medical School, 80
Cornell University, 26
Coronary artery bypass grafting, 54–55
Coronary artery stenting, 137
Cost of health care: administrative costs
    in, 113–15; under Affordable Care Act,
    149; co-pays in, 126, 168; deductibles
    in, 168; and digital invoicing, 120–27;
    geographic variability of, 126; in

health assurance–disease insurance
    approach, 160–63; McKinsey report
    on, 114–15; as percentage of GDP,
    108; vs. quality, focus on, 94–95; in
    rational system, 148; in Universal
    Workers' Compensation Insurance,
    168–69. *See also* Fee structures
"Cost plus" agreements, 54
Council of Europe, 45, 82
Craige, Ernest, *143*
CROs. *See* Contracted research
    organizations
Curbside consults, 39, 101, 177–78
Current Procedural Terminology (CPT),
    121, 124
"Customary and usual" fee structures,
    53, 121, 124, 126

Darling, Helen, 97
Dartmouth College, 22
Davidson, Charles, 40
Decision making: clinical trials and,
    105–6; computers in, 135, 138;
    humanistic, 6; limits of certainty in,
    6; by patients at home, 5
Deductibles, 168
Defined benefit insurance plans, 160–63
Defined contribution insurance plans,
    160–63, 168
Deming, W. Edwards, 94–96
Denham, Charles, 96–97
Denny-Brown, Derek, 40
Devices, licensing of, 106–7, 129, 172
Diabetes, type 2, 7
Dietary Supplement Health and Educa-
    tion Act, 110
Dietary supplements, 109–10
Disease-Related Groups (DRGs),
    121–22, 124
Diseases. *See* Illness; *specific types*
Distress, idioms of, 6, 7, 31
Doctor(s): evolution of meaning of term,
    1, 3; medical, 1, 3; nonmedical, 1.
    See also Physicians

"Doctor, His Patient, and the Illness, The" (Balint), 30–31

Doctor-patient relationship: cultural differences in, 2, 73; electronic records in, 128, 134–35, 138; evolution of roles and rules in, 2–3; guideposts for, 177–80; industrialization of medicine and, 76–77, 108; institutionalization of medicine and, 52; in Japan, 72–73; medical humanism in, 3–15; temporal differences in, 2; trustworthiness in, 5–6, 7; in Universal Workers' Compensation Insurance scheme, 175–76

Dogma, 177–78

DRGs. *See* Disease-Related Groups

Drugs. *See* Clinical trials; Pharmaceutical industry

Duke HealthCare System, 119

Duke University, 99, 103

Dzau, Victor, 99

Ebert, Robert, 35–36

Eclectic Medical College, 22

Eclectic medicine, 20–22

Econometrics, 115

Economies of scale: in group practice, 150; in medical centers, 112–13

Economy, U.S.: cost of health care as percentage of GDP, 108; employment in health-care industry, 112

Education, medical, 32–50; clinical (*See* Clinical education); conflicts of interest in, 98–99, 102; continuing (*See* Continuing Medical Education); with duration of three vs. four years, 138–39; eclectic, 20–22; ethics in, 38; European approach to, 33–34; humanism in, 11–14; Japanese approach to, 71–74; liberal arts tradition and, 32–33; pedagogical flaws of, 34–37; postwar expansion of, 60; preclinical curriculum in,

34–37, 60, 62; premedical classes and, 33; quantifying competency in, 140–44, *142*, *143*; residency training in, 42–46, 49. *See also specific schools*

Education, undergraduate, 32–33

Effectiveness: comparative, research on, 129–32; vs. efficacy, 130; in health assurance–disease insurance approach, 162–63; in Universal Workers' Compensation Insurance scheme, 169–76

Efficacy: vs. effectiveness, 130; in licensing of drugs, 104–7, 129–30; in Universal Workers' Compensation Insurance scheme, 170–73

Efficacy Reviews, 170–73

Efficiency, sacrificing care for, 138–40

EHR. *See* Electronic Health Record

Elderly patients, overtreatment of, 92–93. *See also* Medicare

Electronic Health Record (EHR), 120, 124–27, 128–29, 137

Electronic Medical Record (EMR), 120

Electronic records: coding in, 121–24; and comparative effectiveness research, 129–32; and curbside consults, 177–78; and digital invoicing, 120–27; doctor-patient relationship changed by, 128, 134–35, 138; granularity of data in, 96, 123–26, 129–30; introduction of, 120, 124, 128–29; software for, 132–37; subliminal marketing in, 137–38; subsidies for, 133

Employee Retirement Income Security Act (ERISA), 161

Employment, in health-care industry, 112

EMR. *See* Electronic Medical Record

Engelsher, Charles L., 18–19, 22, 29

Engelsher, Zangwill, 18–19

Engineering, industrial, 94–96

EPIC, 132–37

Erikson, Erik, 15

Errors, medical, 89–92; approaches to reducing, 89–92; definition of, 89, 90; difficulty of measuring, 91, 94; at hospitals, 89–92; in Libby Zion case, 85; overtreatment as, 92–93; rates of, 89, 90; subjectivity in, 91, 94, 95

Ether, 19–20, 43

Ethical issues: AMA Code of Medical Ethics, 53; centrality to medicine, 38; in medical education, 38. *See also* Conflicts of interest

Europe: limits on hours worked in, 45–46, 81–82; medical school curriculum in, 33–34; models of medicine in, 46–47

Evaluation/Management Services (E/M), 121

Faulkner, Judith, 132

Federman, Daniel, 62

Fee structures: co-pays in, 126, 168; "cost plus" agreements in, 54; "customary and usual," 53, 121, 124, 126; in digital invoicing, 120–27; fee-for-service, 18, 27, 56, 61, 70, 120, 121, 176; fees for serving, 175–76; of Medicare, 53–55, 121, 124, 125; sliding scale, 53; in Universal Workers' Compensation Insurance scheme, 174–75

Feinstein, Alvan, 162

Fellowships, 71

Final Determination, 173–74

Finland, Maxwell, 40

Fitz, Reginald, 47

Flexner, Abraham, 21–22, 34, 60

Food, Drug and Cosmetic Act, Kefauver-Harris Amendment to, 8, 104

Food and Drug Administration (FDA): conflicts of interest in, 98, 105; and dietary supplements, 110; funding of, 105; licensing of devices by, 106–7, 129, 172; licensing of drugs by, 104–7, 129, 172; and translational research, 102, 103

Ford Foundation, 24

"Four Laws of Therapeutic Dynamics," 111, 177

French medicine, 46

"From Illness as Culture to Caregiving as Moral Experience" (Kleinman), 156

Frontal lobotomy, 38

GDP. *See* Gross Domestic Product

General Electric, 95, 99

Georgetown Medical School, 62–63

Georgetown University, 113

Gibson, Rosemary, 97–98

Golden, Robert, 98

Goldwater Memorial Hospital, 23–27

Granularity of data, 96, 123–26, 129–30

Gross Domestic Product (GDP), cost of health care as percentage of, 108

Group practice, 150–52

Guideline panels, conflicts of interest in, 98

Guideposts, for future physicians, 177–80

Harvard Medical School: clinical clerkships at, 37–42; humanism at, 12, 14; preclinical curriculum at, 35–36

Hastings Center, 98

Healing movements, sectarian, 20–21

Health: vs. absence of disease, 109; commodification of, 3, 145; as coping with illness, 178–79; evolution of definition of, 3; social construction of, 3, 4, 5, 7, 73; socioeconomic disparities in, 52, 109–10

Health Affairs (journal), 94

Health and Human Services, Department of, 90, 149

Health assurance–disease insurance model, 160–63, 168

Health care: continuity of, 81–84; cost of (*See* Cost of health care);

disparities in access to, 52; industrialization of, 76–77; outcomes of, limits on physician hours and, 46, 82–85; quality of (*See* Quality of care); rationing of, 161; universal access to, 147

Health Care Blog, The (THCB), 130–32

Health Care Financing Administration (HCFA), 78

Health Care Quality Innovation Fund, 89–90

Health-care system, Japanese, 72–73

Health-care system, U.S.: consolidation of businesses in, 112–20; doctor-patient relationship changed by, 2–3; employment in sector, 112; humanism of, as measure of success, 7; industrialization of, 76–77, 108; rational alternative to, 147–49

Health Information Technology for Economic and Clinical Health (HI TECH), 132–33

Health insurance: defined benefit plans, 160–63; defined contribution plans, 160–63, 168; doctor-patient relationship affected by, 2–3; health assurance–disease insurance approach to, 160–63, 168; Medicare fee structure used in, 54; rise of, in 1970s, 54; workers' compensation insurance as model for, 164–75

Health Insurance Portability and Accountability Act (HIPAA) of 1996, 39–40

Health savings accounts (HSAs), 168

Heart attacks, 137

Herz, Marcus, 11

Hill-Burton Act. *See* Hospital Survey and Construction Act

HIPAA. *See* Health Insurance Portability and Accountability Act

Hippocrates, 23

Hippocratic Oath, 10

Homeopathic medicine, 20–22

Hospital(s): administration of, in 1970s, 56, 63–64; bed-rest cure in, 22–23; business models of, 112–20; duration of stays at, 23, 100; medical errors at, 89–92; medical school–affiliated, 17, 24 (*See also* Teaching hospitals); municipal, 17, 22, 27–29; postwar construction of, 60, 112; proprietary, 17–20, 22–23, 28, 31; regional medical centers replacing, 112–14; voluntary, 18. *See also specific hospitals*

Hospitalists, 22, 83

Hospital Survey and Construction Act (Hill-Burton Act), 112, 114

HSAs. *See* Health savings accounts

Hsiao, William, 124

Humanism, medical, 1–15; in clinical education, 11–14; in decision making, 6; definition of, 3–4, 6; evolution of, 4, 6; in France, 46; in nineteenth century, 11–13; and religion, 9–11; return to ideal of, 156; and symptoms of unknown origin, 13–14

Hume, David, 105

Hutchison, Robert, 147–48

Idioms of distress, 6, 7, 31

Illness: absence of, vs. health, 109; coping with, 178–80; evolution of definition of, 3; as injury, 166; patient's experience of, 4–6; as product line, 3, 77, 145; social construction of, 3, 4, 5; terminal, overtreatment of, 92–93

Imperturbability, 11

Industrial engineering, 94–96

Industrialization, of medicine, 76–77, 108

Ingbar, Sidney, 40

Injuries: back, 165–66; broadening definition of, 166–67; in workers' compensation, 164–67

Inpatient care. *See* Hospital(s)

Institute for Healthcare Improvement (IHI), 96, 99
Institute of Medicine, 89–90, 98, 99, 139, 161
Institutionalization of medicine, 52, 175
Insurance. *See* Health insurance; Workers' compensation
Intensive Care Units (ICU), overuse of, 92–93
International Statistical Classification of Diseases and Related Health Problems (ICD), 122–24, 125
Invincibility, sense of, 179
Invoicing: digital, 120–27; in Universal Workers' Compensation Insurance, 174–75. *See also* Fee structures

Jandl, James, 40
Japan: clinical education in, 71–74; health-care system of, 72–73
Jefferson Medical College, 60
Johns Hopkins Medical School, 11–12, 34, 41, 133
Johnson, Lyndon, 52–53, 120
Journal of the American Medical Association, 12, 98, 140
Judgment: in effectiveness determinations, 173–74; in efficacy reviews, 170–73; and medical errors, 91; surgical, 39
Justice, Department of, 78–79, 96

Kaiser Foundation Health Plans and Hospitals, 97
Kaiser Health System, 133
Kaiser-Permanente, 153
Kant, Immanuel, 11
Kefauver-Harris Amendment, 8, 104
Kelley, William, 113
King, John, 21
Kleinman, Arthur, 31, 156
Knowledge, profound, 95–96
Knowledge of Man, The (Buber), 157
Kyoto University, 74

Labels, for symptoms of unknown origin, 13–14
Lancet, The (journal), 30
Lanza, Joseph "Socks," 18
Lasagna, Louis, 32
Leape, Lucian, 90–91, 94
"Libby Zion Law" (New York), 81, 84–85
Liberal arts tradition, 32–33
Licensing, of devices, 106–7, 129, 172
Licensing, of drugs, 104–7; conflicts of interest in, 105–7; efficacy in, 104–7, 129–30; problems with criteria for, 104–7; in Universal Workers' Compensation Insurance scheme, 172
Licensing, of physicians: in early — twentieth century, 18, 22; physician control of, 53
Lipkin, Mack, 9
Listening, 26, 179–80
Literature, medical: anecdotal, 8; in efficacy reviews, 171–72; meta-analyses of, 106, 107
Lobotomy, frontal, 38
Locums practitioners, 82–83
London, Tavistock Clinic in, 30

MacArthur, Douglas, 94
Maimonides, Moses, 10–11
Maintenance of certification (MOC), 142–44
Maizuru Municipal Hospital, 73–74
Malaria, 24
Malpractice, Type 2 Medical, 92
Management consulting firms, 112–13, 114–15
Mark, Vernon Herschel, 37–39
Marketing, subliminal, 137–38
Massachusetts General Hospital (MGH): "Allen Street" conference at, 45, 66; Baker Pavilion at, 44, 48, 49; Bulfinch Building at, 43–44, 47–49; cardiovascular surgery at, 54–55; clinical education at, 38–40, 67–68; clinical investigation at,

47–48; international reputation of, 47; medical service of, 42–45, 182 (n. 7); as modern teaching hospital, 47–50; Phillips House at, 44, 48, 49; residency training at, 42–46, 49
Massachusetts Medical Society, 14
Matsumura, Tadashi, 72–73, 74
McKinsey and Company, 114–15
McKinsey Global Institute (MGI), 114–15
Medco, 99
Media coverage, of Parkchester General Hospital, 19–20
Medical centers, regional: business models of, 112–20; economies of scale in, 112–13; as major source of employment, 112; rise of, 112–13
Medical homes, 152–53
Medical Malpractice, Type 2, 92
Medicare, 52–56; effect on clinical training, 55–56, 77–79; establishment of, 51, 52–53; fee structure of, 53–55, 121, 124, 125; measures of quality of care in, 96; medical errors under, 90; variability of charges to, 126–27
Medtronic, 99
Mendelssohn, Moses, 11
Merck, 59
Meta-analyses, 106, 107
Metabolic syndrome, 7
Metrics, overemphasis on, 4–5
Metropolitan Life Insurance Company (MetLife), 16
Meymandi, Assad, 10–11
Middlesex Medical School, 20–22
Military service: commissioned public health officers as alternative to, 56–57; veterans of, 30
Mill, John Stuart, 105
Minot, George, 40
Mississippi, workers' compensation in, 164
Mitchell, Silas Weir, 22–23

Montefiore Hospital, 28
Morbidity. *See* Illness
Moreland Act of 1907 (New York), 18
Morgenthau, Robert, 81
"Morning Prayer of the Physician, The," 9–11, 15, 139, 147
Morris, Gouverneur, 27
Morris, Lewis, 27
Morrisania Hospital, 27–29
Motorola Corporation, 95
Mount Vernon Daily Argus (newspaper), 18
Multispecialty practice, 150–52
MUMPS (Multi-User Multi-Programming System), 132
Municipal hospitals, in 1950s, 17, 22, 27–29. *See also specific hospitals*
Murphy, William, 40

National Academies Press, 161
National Academy of Sciences, 89–91
National Academy of Social Insurance, 167
National Institutes of Health (NIH): Clinical Center at, 47, 56–58; and clinical education, 62–63; commissioned public health officers in, 56–57; grants from, 37
National Quality Forum (NQF), 96–97, 99
National Science Foundation, 37
Neuroleptic malignant syndrome, 80, 85, 87
Neurosurgery, 37–38
New England Journal of Medicine, 14, 156
New Jersey, workers' compensation in, 164
New York: "Libby Zion Law" in, 81, 84–85; workers' compensation in, 164
New York City, hospitals of 1950s in, 17–29
New York Hospital, Libby Zion's death at, 79–81, 85–88

New York State Department of
Health, 81
New York State Hospital
Commission, 17
New York Times (newspaper), 19, 80
Night float rotation, 83, 84
NIH. *See* National Institutes of Health
NNT. *See* Number Needed to Treat
North Carolina Memorial Hospital, 60,
63, 86
Not-for-profit companies, 114, 118
"Not the Disease Only, but Also the
Man" (Putnam), 14
Number Needed to Treat (NNT), 104
Nurses: charge, 66, 68; locums
(short-term), 83

Obama, Barack, 90, 129
Obamacare. *See* Affordable Care Act
Obesity, 109
Occupational diseases, 165
Osler, William: "Aequanimitas," 2, 11,
181 (n. 1); humanism of, 11–12, 14
Outpatient care: under Affordable Care
Act, 149; cost of, 115; at freestanding
specialist clinics, 101, 151; in group
and multispecialty practice, 150–52;
at patient-centered clinics, 152;
teaching of, 64–65. *See also* Private
practice
Overtreatment, 92–93, 148
Overweight, 109

Pain: back, and workers' compensation,
165–66; coping with, 179–80
Parkchester General Hospital, 17–20,
22–23
Parkchester neighborhood, 16–17
Patient(s): coping with illness, 178–80;
decision making at home by, 5;
experience of illness, 4–6; outcomes
of, limits on physician hours and,
46, 82–85; psychosocial challenges
facing ill, 2–3; safety of, 89, 90–91,

94; transition back from patient to
person, 75–76; as units of care, 77,
119–20, 145, 178
Patient-centered clinics, 152
Patient-Centered Outcomes Research
Institute (PCORI), 130–32
Payer, Lynne, 71–72
"Pay-for-performance," 96, 97, 153–54
Peabody, Francis Weld, 12–14, 40
Peer review, of clinical competence,
69, 140
Pennsylvania Chronic Care Initiative,
154–55
PepsiCo, 99
Performance, pay for, 96, 97, 153–54
Pharmaceutical industry: conflicts of
interest in, 59, 101–2, 105–7; in
Continuing Medical Education, 59;
licensing of drugs and, 104–7.
See also Clinical trials
Physicians: evolution of term, 1; guide-
posts for future, 177–80; limits on
hours worked by, 45–46, 79–89; as
master clinicians, 157; Medicare's
effects on role of, 52–55; retirement
of, 151; trustworthiness as prereq-
uisite for, 5–6, 7. *See also* Attending
physicians; Doctor-patient relation-
ship; Specialists
Pisano, Etta, 98–99
Plain Language Summary, 173–74
Popper, Karl, 105
PPD, 103
Preclinical education, 34–37, 60, 62
Premedical education, 33
Premier, Inc., 97
Premiums: in Universal Workers'
Compensation Insurance scheme,
168–69; in workers' compensation,
165
Private hospitals. *See* Proprietary
hospitals
Private practice: in 1970s and 1980s, 58;
bought by hospitals, 113; business

model of, 58, 117, 150–52; decline of, 113, 117; vs. group practice, 150

Procedures, lack of licensing of, 129

Productivity, industrial approaches to increasing, 94–96

Professionalism, medical, 159–76; clinical education in acquisition of, 85; curbside consults in, 178; dynamics of, 3; guideposts for, 177–80; in health assurance–disease insurance model, 160–63, 168; modeling of, 140; in workers' compensation model, 164–76

Profound knowledge, 95–96

Proprietary hospitals: in 1950s, 17–20, 22–23, 28; decline and return of, 31

ProPublica, 97

"Providers," physicians as, 178

Prussian medicine, 46–47

Psychoanalysis, 30–31

Psychological disorders, in veterans, 30

Psychosocial challenges, facing ill patients, 2–3

Psychosurgery, 38

Public health officers, commissioned, 56–57

Putnam, James J., 14

Quality and Outcomes Framework, 154

Quality of care: conflicts of interest in evaluation of, 96–99; vs. cost, focus on, 94–95; growth of industry for measuring, 96; limits on physician hours and, 82, 84; problems with metrics for, 4–5; "systems" approach to, 89, 90, 94

Quality of Health Care in America Committee, 89–90

Quintiles Transnational, 103

Rabelais, 46

RAND Corporation, 125–26, 154

Randomized controlled trials (RCTs), 104–7, 129–30

Rationality: in health care, 147–49, 157; in health insurance, 160–63, 164; in Universal Workers' Compensation Insurance, 175–76

Rationing of health care, 161

RBRVS Update Committee (RUC), 124

RCTs. See Randomized controlled trials

Record keeping: and digital invoicing, 120–27; paper, 128–29, 135–36. See also Electronic records

Reductionist science, 11–13

Refutationist science, 105

Regional medical centers. See Medical centers

Regulatory capture, 124–25

Religion: and health promotion, 110; and medical humanism, 9–11

Relman, Arnold, 156

Residency training: limits on hours worked in, 45–46, 79–89; Medicare's effects on, 77–79; at teaching hospitals in 1960s, 42–46, 49

Resource-Based Relative Value Scale (RBRVS), 124

Retirement, physician, 151

Rex Hospital, 119

Reynolds, Malvina, 117

Risk: relative vs. absolute reduction of, 106; shared, 162

Robert Wood Johnson Foundation, 98

Roosevelt, Theodore, 157

Royal College of Surgeons, 82

Rural areas, hospitals in, 112

Safety, patient: checklists for, 90–91; difficulty of measuring, 94; "systems" approach to, 89, 90, 94

Schactman, Fred, 30

Schools, medical. See Education; *specific schools*

Schweitzer, Laura, 98

Science: in medical school curriculum, 33–35; reductionist, 11–13; refutationist, 105; in undergraduate studies, 33

Science Honors Program (Columbia University), 24
Scribes, 128, 135
Sectarian healing movements, 20–21
Seed trials, 103
Seegal, Beatrice Carrier, 24–25, 32
Seegal, David, 24–26, *25*, 29, 32, 177
Seeger, Pete, 117
Selby, Joe, 130–32
Serotonin syndrome, 80, 85, 87
SES. *See* Socioeconomic status
Shannon, James, 24
Shared risk, 162
Shattuck Lecture, 14
Sherman, Raymond, 80, 85–86
"Six sigma" approach, 95
Sliding scale, 53
Smith, Bill, 94–95
Social construction: of back injuries, 166; of health and illness, 3, 4, 5, 7, 73
"Socialized medicine," 53
Social Security Act, Title XVIII of. *See* Medicare
Socioeconomic status (SES): and Body Mass Index, 109; and disparities in health, 52, 109–10
Software, health-care, 132–37
Specialists: and definition of "physician," 1; freestanding clinics of, 101, 151; in group practice, 150–51; rise of, 69–70; subspecialization by, 1, 70; at teaching hospitals, 70–71, 100–101
Statistical significance, 104–5
Stead, Eugene, 36–37
Steinman, Ralph, 36
STEMI, 137
Stimulus bill. *See* American Recovery and Reinvestment Act
Stock market crash of 1929, 16
Stone, Greg, 80
Subsidies, for electronic records, 133
Subspecialization: in clinical education, 70–71; rise of, 1, 70

Supplements, dietary, 109–10
Supreme Court, U.S., 164
Surgeons: in 1960s, education of, 37–40; in 1970s and 1980s, education of, 65–66; in early twentieth century, regulation of, 18–20; specialization of, 69–70
Surgery: cardiovascular, rise of, 54–55; licensing of devices in, 106–7; medical errors in, 90–91
Surgical judgment, 39
Symptoms of unknown origin, humanism for patients with, 13–14
"Systems" approach, 89, 90, 94

Tavistock Clinic, 30
Teaching hospitals: closure of, 113; conflicts of interest in, 107; creation of modern, in 1960s, 47–50; erosion of role in clinical education, 75–79; fragmentation of patient care in, 81–84, 99–100; growth of, in 1970s, 51–52, 60; Japanese, 71–74; limits on hours worked in, 45–46, 79–89; Medicare's effects on, 55–56, 77–79; residency training in 1960s at, 42–46, 49; specialists and subspecialists at, 70–71, 100–101; translational research at, 103. *See also* Clinical education; *specific institutions*
Technion-Israel Institute of — Technology, 26
Terminal illnesses, overtreatment of, 92–93
Thomas, Lewis, 9
Thorndike Memorial Laboratory, 12, 40
"Thought leaders," 103, 107, 137
"Three-legged stools," 57, 60, 61
Time magazine, 36
"To Err Is Human" report, 89–91, 94, 98
"Training for Tomorrow's Needs" (essay), 36
Translational research, 102–4, 107
Trials. *See* Clinical trials

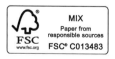